KETO FITNESS COOKBOOK

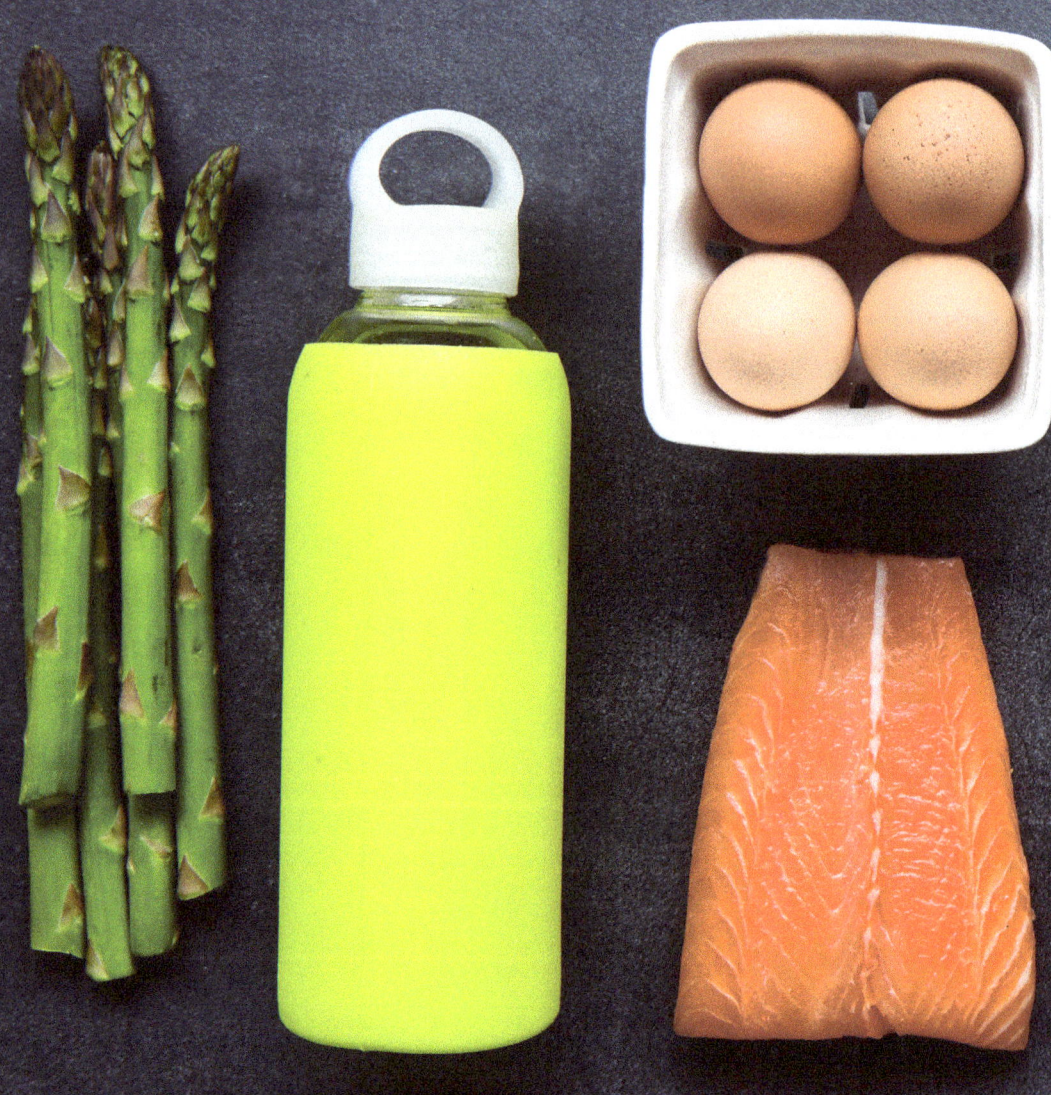

KETO FITNESS COOKBOOK

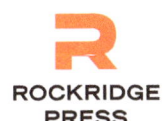

RECIPES AND MEAL PLANS TO MAXIMIZE YOUR WORKOUTS

Molly Devine, RD

R
ROCKRIDGE PRESS

For my husband, my fitness and all-around awesome life partner.

Copyright © 2021 by Rockridge Press, Emeryville, California

No part of this publication may be reproduced, stored in a retrieval system, or transmitted in any form or by any means, electronic, mechanical, photocopying, recording, scanning, or otherwise, except as permitted under Sections 107 or 108 of the 1976 United States Copyright Act, without the prior written permission of the Publisher. Requests to the Publisher for permission should be addressed to the Permissions Department, Rockridge Press, 6005 Shellmound Street, Suite 175, Emeryville, CA 94608.

Limit of Liability/Disclaimer of Warranty: The Publisher and the author make no representations or warranties with respect to the accuracy or completeness of the contents of this work and specifically disclaim all warranties, including without limitation warranties of fitness for a particular purpose. No warranty may be created or extended by sales or promotional materials. The advice and strategies contained herein may not be suitable for every situation. This work is sold with the understanding that the Publisher is not engaged in rendering medical, legal, or other professional advice or services. If professional assistance is required, the services of a competent professional person should be sought. Neither the Publisher nor the author shall be liable for damages arising herefrom. The fact that an individual, organization, or website is referred to in this work as a citation and/or potential source of further information does not mean that the author or the Publisher endorses the information the individual, organization, or website may provide or recommendations they/it may make. Further, readers should be aware that websites listed in this work may have changed or disappeared between when this work was written and when it is read.

For general information on our other products and services or to obtain technical support, please contact our Customer Care Department within the United States at (866) 744-2665, or outside the United States at (510) 253-0500.

Rockridge Press publishes its books in a variety of electronic and print formats. Some content that appears in print may not be available in electronic books, and vice versa.

TRADEMARKS: Rockridge Press and the Rockridge Press logo are trademarks or registered trademarks of Callisto Media Inc. and/or its affiliates, in the United States and other countries, and may not be used without written permission. All other trademarks are the property of their respective owners. Rockridge Press is not associated with any product or vendor mentioned in this book.

Interior and Cover Designer: Rachel Haeseker
Art Producer: Sue Bischofberger
Editor: Maxine Marshall

Photography © Annie Martin, cover, pp vi, 48; Marija Vidal, pp ii, 2, 58; Laura Flippen, pp viii, 1; Nadine Greeff, pp 16, 104; Darren Muir, pp 26, 80; Helene Dujardin, pp 46, 47; Evi Abeler, p. 68; Emulsion Studio, p. 94; Biz Jones, p. 114. Author photograph courtesy of Heba Salama Photography

ISBN: Print 978-1-64876-894-1
eBook 978-1-64876-895-8

R0

CONTENTS

Introduction vii

PART 1
The Keto-Fit Program 1

CHAPTER 1
Powering Up with the Ketogenic Diet 3

CHAPTER 2
Inside the Keto-Fit Kitchen 17

CHAPTER 3
Keto-Fit Meal Plans 27

PART 2
Keto-Fit Recipes 47

CHAPTER 4
Breakfast 49

CHAPTER 5
Vegetables and Sides 59

CHAPTER 6
Seafood and Poultry 69

CHAPTER 7
Pork and Beef 81

CHAPTER 8
Snacks and Staples 95

CHAPTER 9
Desserts 105

Measurement Conversions 115
References 116
Index 118

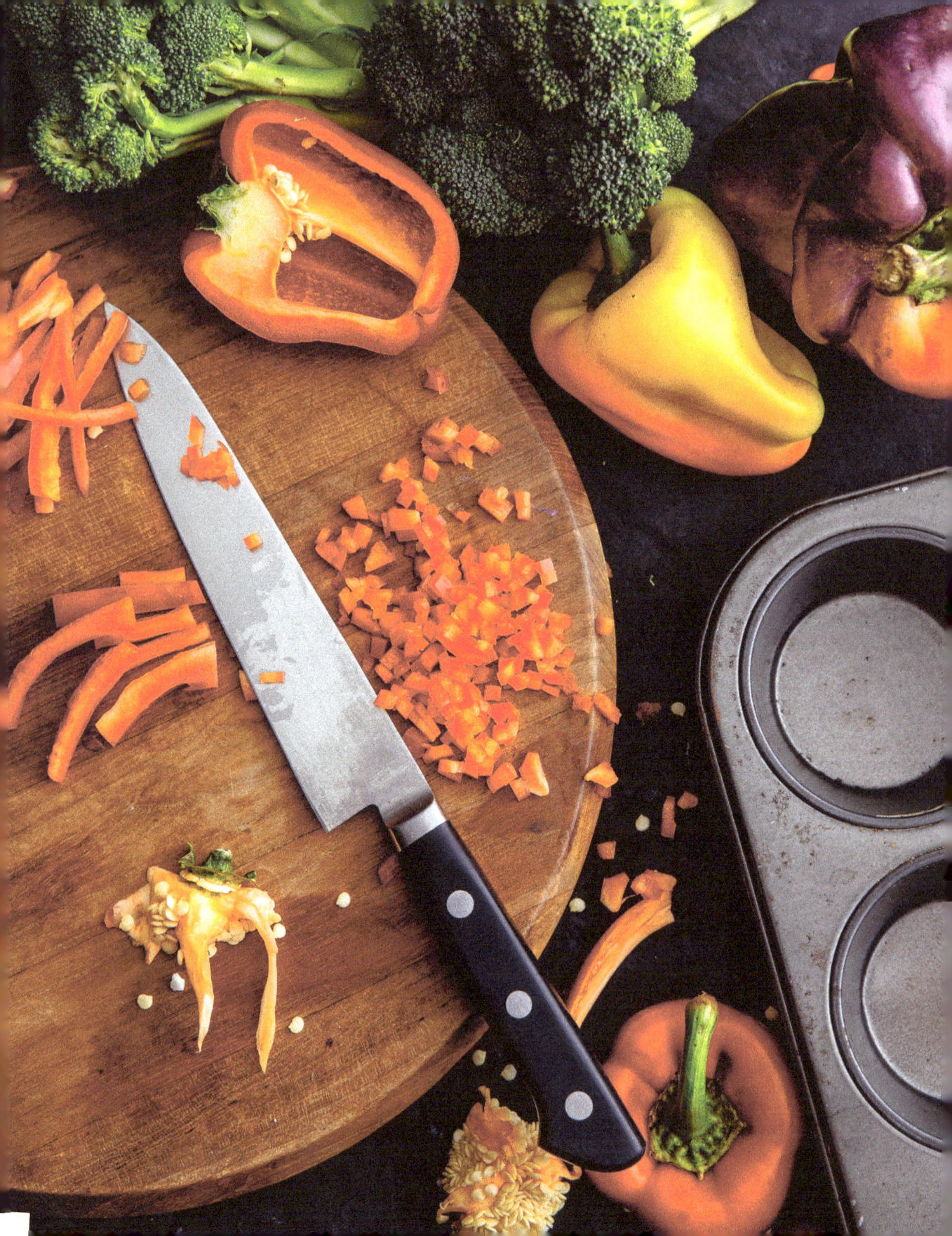

INTRODUCTION

ALTHOUGH PHYSICAL ACTIVITY AND EXERCISE are important to overall health, you can't outrun a poor diet! As a registered dietitian specializing in integrative and functional nutrition, I help my clients understand that food is our best medicine and that proper nutrition is the cornerstone to optimal health, performance, and healthy weight maintenance. A well-formulated dietary intervention can drastically improve the way we feel, inside and out. Although nutrition is about 70 to 80 percent of the puzzle, it is also imperative to pay attention to other lifestyle factors, such as stress, sleep, and physical activity, to really create a complete wheel of health. Allowing our nutrition to fuel our busy and active lifestyles supports a symbiotic relationship among all health factors.

In recent years, the ketogenic dietary approach has gained significant popularity for its health benefits, which include weight management, decreased inflammation, improved blood sugar control, and increased energy. All of these positive outcomes contribute directly to athletic performance. Truly understanding the basics of a balanced ketogenic diet can be a game changer for athletes and for people who are looking for a variety of health benefits from physical activity beyond just shedding pounds.

As a lifelong competitive swimmer, I have seen firsthand how a ketogenic way of eating can improve body composition, increase endurance, and provide sustainable fuel through longer workouts. However, it is crucial to have all the necessary tools when starting this dietary intervention for athletic performance, including proper guidance, reasonable expectations, sustainable meal plans, and quick and easy recipes. That is why I wrote this book! By bringing together two elements I feel very passionate about—healthy, whole foods–based ketogenic nutrition plans and exercise—in an easy-to-understand way, I hope to help you achieve your fitness goals while also improving and sustaining a balanced, healthy lifestyle.

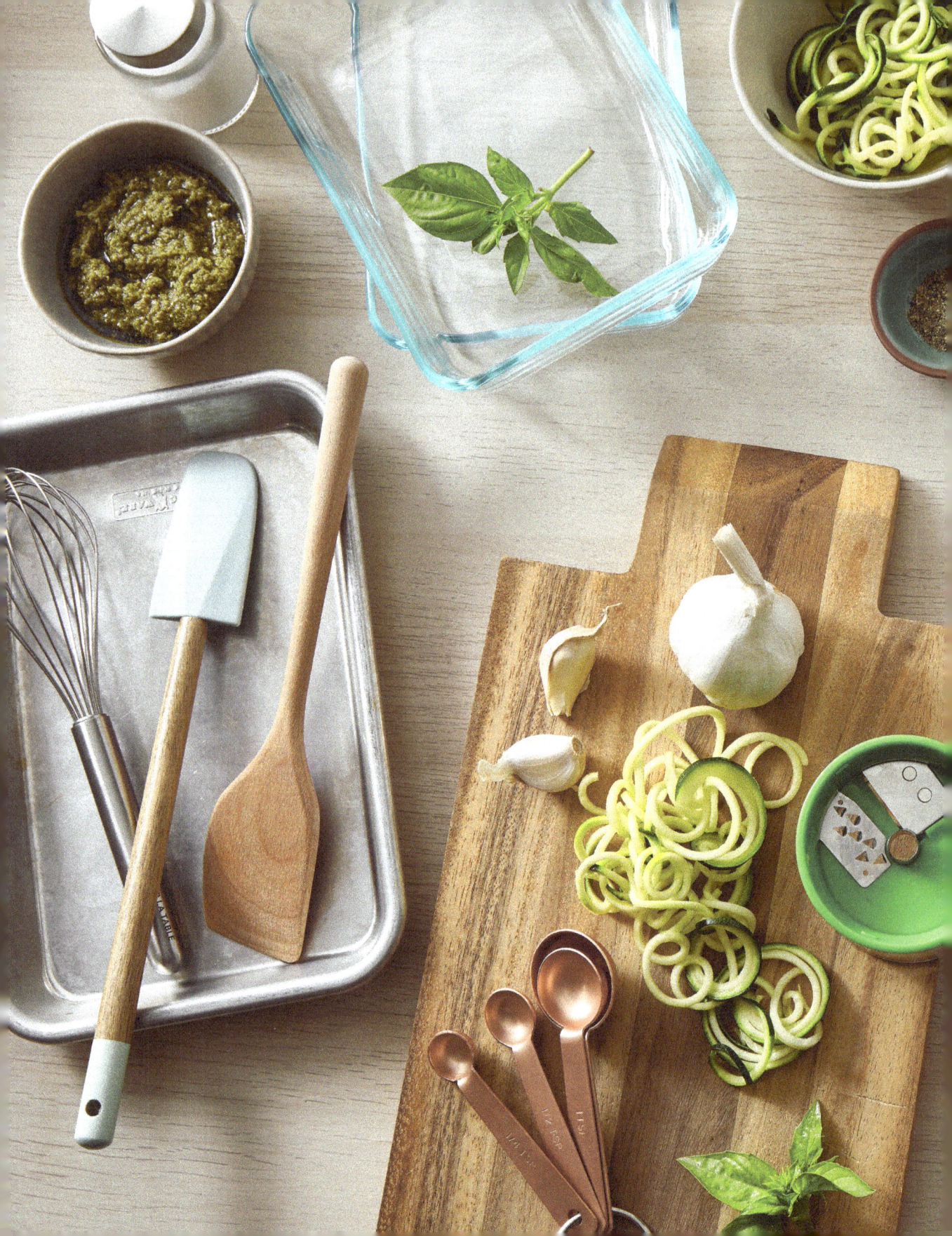

PART 1
THE KETO-FIT PROGRAM

NUTRITION EDUCATION CAN EMPOWER YOU with the knowledge you need for long-term success, enabling you to make keto a lifestyle rather than just another diet. Understanding your body's needs, especially related to exercise, will help you feel more connected to the process and provide motivation to continue toward your goals. Before we dive into the recipes, we'll establish that foundational knowledge. I like to think of the first chapter of this book as "Keto Fitness 101," because it is designed to get you up to speed on everything you need to know about the powerful combination of exercise and the ketogenic diet. Chapter 2 covers what foods to include on your plate and the necessary tools for easy meal prep. In chapter 3, I lay out four different one-week meal plans for a variety of workout regimens and weight goals, along with shopping lists and prep tips to get the ball rolling.

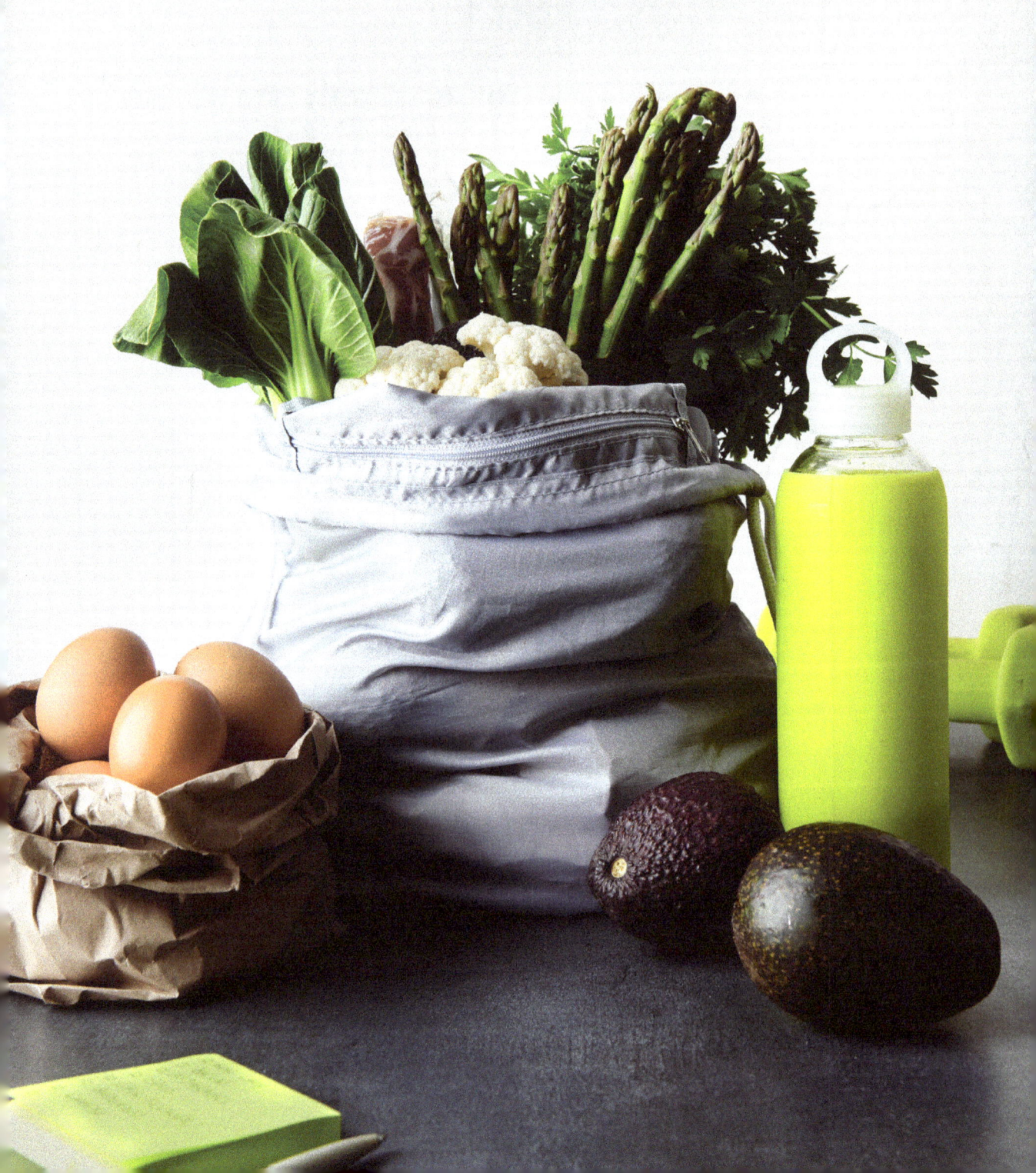

CHAPTER 1

Powering Up with the Ketogenic Diet

WHETHER YOU ARE NEW TO KETO OR AN OLD PRO, understanding how it relates to physical fitness and how to time meals around your workout routine is key to reaping all the benefits of a keto-fit nutrition plan. This chapter covers the basics of a ketogenic diet and discusses how to customize this approach to achieve your fitness goals.

Achieving Your Fitness Goals with the Help of Keto

No matter what your fitness goals may be, from beginner to seasoned athlete, implementing a ketogenic approach to your nutrition plan may help you augment your progress. Although a ketogenic diet is a well-known approach for weight loss, this way of eating, when formulated correctly for your body's needs, can also help you maintain a healthy weight while losing excess body fat, growing lean body mass, and overall improving body composition. Simply put, being an athlete in a state of ketosis does not mean constantly losing weight, and it can lead to heightened performance, endurance, and strength.

As you will read in greater detail in the sections that follow, a ketogenic diet restricts most carbohydrates (which come from sugars, grains, starchy vegetables, and many higher-sugar fruits), but it is filled with satiating, flavorful, and fun foods. A healthy keto diet sources protein from meats, fish, poultry, dairy, and eggs, as well as healthy fats from avocados, oils, nuts, seeds, and fatty fish. You'll also enjoy fiber-rich and nutrient-dense carbohydrates from green leafy and non-starchy vegetables to add color and bulk to each meal. I always encourage my clients to approach any dietary plan from a "glass half full" mentality: Focus on what you get to include on your plate, not what to take off. This balanced approach to a ketogenic way of eating, along with the easy and flavorful recipes and meal plans that follow, make this lifestyle enjoyable, sustainable, and never boring!

It is important to cater your nutrition plan to your level of activity and lifestyle, which is why a customized approach is key to success no matter what your goals. In the following sections, I will help you understand not only the ins and outs of a ketogenic diet and why it works, but also how to use this metabolic process to your advantage for a variety of different exercise routines and activity levels. Timing and portions will be dependent on exercise type and intensity.

The Fitness Benefits of the Keto Diet

A whole foods–based ketogenic diet offers many benefits to people who exercise frequently or who are trying to improve athletic performance.

Protein-Sparing Weight Loss: Ketones are a protein-sparing fuel source. When you are nourished with a diet including adequate protein, nutritional ketosis promotes body fat loss while preserving lean body mass and muscle. This is especially true when a ketogenic diet is combined with intermittent fasting or fasted workouts (see page 13).

Increased Endurance: After a period of nutritional ketosis, the body seamlessly uses stored fat for energy. Fat is a more efficient energy source than glucose at 9 calories per gram versus 4 calories per gram. Furthermore, muscular athletes can only store 1,000 to 1,800 calories worth of glycogen energy (about 15g/kg of body weight) for use during exercise. Compared to potential energy storage from fat, this is a drop in the bucket.

Improved Cognitive Function: When the body is in ketosis, the brain utilizes ketones, a more efficient fuel source than glucose, leading to better focus during sports and the mental capacity to power through challenging workouts.

Blood Sugar Control: Studies show that a ketogenic diet reduces fluctuations in blood sugar and insulin. Not only does this lower your risk of developing insulin resistance and type 2 diabetes, but also this prevents blood sugar drops after longer workouts.

Decreased Risk for Injury: A diet high in refined carbohydrates, sugars, and poor-quality fats like processed vegetable oils leads to fluid retention, joint swelling, and pain, leaving us ripe for injury. Conversely, a whole foods–based keto diet provides our bodies with the omega-3 fatty acids (found in fish, nuts, and seeds) needed to create anti-inflammatory mediators. These mediators turn off inflammation in the body, supporting recovery and injury prevention.

Why the Keto Diet Works

A properly formulated ketogenic diet is more complex than being simply "low carb." The majority of energy, or calories, consumed on a keto diet needs to come from dietary fat, while only a moderate amount needs to come from protein (just enough to support individual needs) and a very low amount from carbohydrates. This allows the body to convert from a "glucose burn" (from the breakdown of carbohydrates) to a "fat burn" (from the breakdown of fatty acids) mode, relying on both dietary fat sources and stored body fat for energy. This is the metabolic state of *ketosis*, from which the ketogenic diet derives its name.

Not all cells can use pure fatty acids for fuel, and most importantly, the brain cannot use them at all. Ketosis is the body's process of converting these fatty acids into usable currency for energy: a ketone. Fatty acids travel to the liver, where they are converted into ketones and sent throughout the body for use as energy. Ketones are like rocket fuel; they are extremely efficient, provide long-term energy, and improve function, making them an ideal fuel source for many endurance activities.

The ability to achieve and maintain ketosis is different for everyone and varies based on previous carbohydrate intake, body composition, insulin resistance, and fitness routine. But generally, the ketogenic ratios and meal plans outlined in this book should allow your body to enter ketosis within 3 or 4 days. When paired with regular exercise, maintaining a state of metabolic ketosis can help accelerate weight loss, improve body composition (you will lose fat while maintaining muscle mass), and provide increased energy and satiety through longer workouts. Additionally, as I will discuss in the following sections, regular exercise combined with intermittent fasting can often allow many individuals to have more flexibility with carbohydrate ratios while remaining ketogenic.

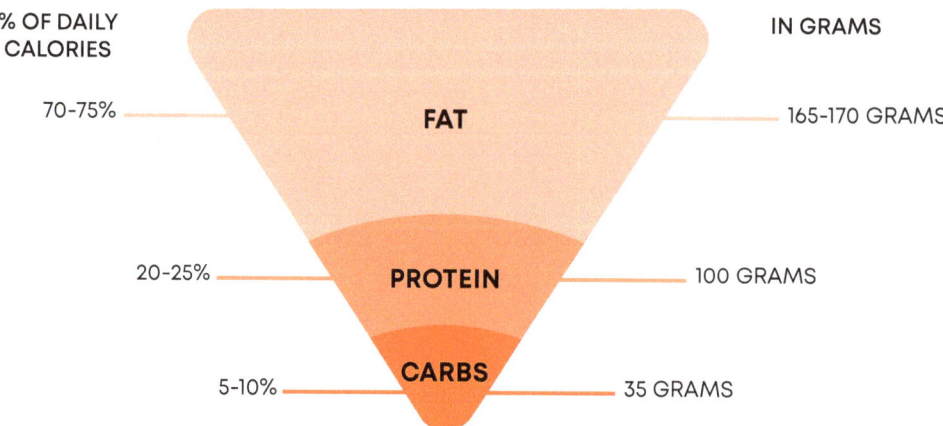

Understanding the Keto Ratio

Macronutrients, or "macros" for short, are the building blocks of our diet. All food breaks down into one of three macronutrients: protein, carbohydrate, and fat, and many foods (such as dairy or nuts) are a combination of two or three. Carbohydrates and proteins provide 4 calories of energy per gram, while fats provide 9 calories of energy per gram. The macro ratio for a standard ketogenic diet is 70 to 75 percent of your daily energy (calories) coming from fat, 20 to 25 percent from protein, and 5 to 10 percent from carbohydrates, but everyone's bodies are different and certain individuals have higher protein needs or can tolerate higher levels of carbohydrate from high-fiber, plant-based sources while remaining ketogenic. A whole foods–based ketogenic diet doesn't have to be boring and is filled with delicious and nutritious options that are typically very affordable!

There are several online resources to calculate your individual macronutrient needs based on age, height, weight, and activity level. If you would like to establish personalized daily targets, I suggest using an app such as MyFitnessPal or Cronometer, both of which have free versions. The meal plans and recipes that follow are designed around a 1,500 to 1,800 daily calorie range, depending on activity level and goal. To adjust this up or down, you can change the serving size of each recipe based on hunger, progress, and individual lifestyle needs.

FAT (70 TO 75 PERCENT OF DAILY CALORIES)

Keto enthusiasts love being able to enjoy rich, satiating foods but sometimes overlook the importance of quality fat choices. A high-fat diet doesn't mean unlimited bacon, butter, cream, and steak. The most beneficial and energizing ketogenic diet is rich in heart-healthy unsaturated fats from plant and marine sources such as nuts and seeds, olive oil, avocados, and fatty fish such as salmon, sardines, and anchovies.

PROTEINS (20 TO 25 PERCENT OF DAILY CALORIES)

One of the biggest differences between a ketogenic diet and a low-carb/high-protein diet is the moderation of protein. That's because our bodies will turn excess protein (and in small amounts, excess fat) into glucose for use as fuel before producing ketones. This process is called gluconeogenesis and is a normal daily process, even for those on a ketogenic diet, because glucose is essential for a number of bodily functions. However, if we eat more protein than the body needs on a regular basis, the body will continue to run on glucose, thus preventing ketosis (fat-burn). Many people overconsume protein, thinking that it only goes to their muscles. In fact, most people cannot absorb more than 25 to 35 grams of protein per meal (4 to 6 ounces of meat or fish). Aside from meat and fish, other great sources of protein on a ketogenic diet include eggs and dairy such as full-fat Greek yogurt and cottage cheese, tofu, and nuts and seeds such as hemp.

CARBOHYDRATES (LESS THAN 10 PERCENT OF DAILY CALORIES)

Prioritize consuming plant-based carbohydrates such as non-starchy vegetables and low-sugar fruits rather than processed keto-friendly packaged food products. The former are chock-full of micronutrients (vitamins and minerals) which are essential for cell function, metabolism, digestion, and overall health. The latter tend to be mostly "filler fibers" that the body cannot process well, plus chemicals and additives such as artificial sweeteners and dyes, and inflammatory fats. For this reason, total carbs, rather than "net carbs" (total carb grams minus fiber grams) is the best number to watch when you are monitoring your carb intake. For maximum health benefit, the carbohydrates in your diet should come primarily from whole-foods sources like dark leafy greens; colorful fruits and vegetables, like bell peppers and berries; and fibers found in nuts and seeds.

How Can I Tell If I'm in Ketosis?

Once your body becomes more efficient at producing and using ketones as its primary fuel source, you'll notice that you feel less hungry and more energetic. You'll experience increased mental clarity, improved sleep, and reduced fluid retention exhibited by a rapid weight loss that levels off after the first week or so. These results are the best indicators of a true state of ketosis. If you want to measure your ketone production in a more "clinical" way, you can do so using either blood ketone meters, breath ketone meters, or urine strips.

Urine strips are the cheapest option of the three and measure the ketones that are excreted in your urine. Urine strips are only effective in the beginning stages of ketosis, before your body begins using ketones effectively. Once you have become more "fat adapted," there is less ketone waste and these strips are not as indicative of a state of ketosis.

To determine how certain exercises and foods may impact your personal ketone levels, consider purchasing a blood ketone meter, many of which also measure glucose levels. Check fasting levels in the morning (before eating), after a workout, and two hours after a ketogenic meal to gather data about how your body responds to various foods and activities. Once you can connect these levels with how your body feels (always the best indicator of success!), it is not necessary to check frequently unless your routine changes, you stop seeing progress, or you start feeling different after workouts.

Breath ketone meters are an even more accurate way to measure ketone production, especially as you become more keto adapted and efficient at using ketones for energy, but they tend to be more pricey. For this reason, I only recommend breath meters for those not seeing results and wanting to have a better way to test sensitivity to foods and exercise.

Exercise and the Keto Diet

Now that you understand the nuts and bolts behind a well-formulated ketogenic diet, the next step is learning how to combine these nutrition principles with your active lifestyle to help you achieve your fitness goals.

Most people experience an adjustment phase as they ease into ketosis, no matter what their activity level, so be patient with yourself and remember that you can always adapt your meal plans to fit the timing and intensity of your workouts. Some activities and workouts are more keto-compatible than others, so the following sections discuss the pros and cons of a keto-fit lifestyle for three different types of exercise: cardio, strength training or HIIT, and stretching/rest. No matter what your goals or activity level, following a ketogenic diet is possible while maintaining high-level performance, keeping in mind that some customization may be necessary.

CARDIO

There are two main types of exercise: aerobic and anaerobic activity. Aerobic is a fancy way of saying "with oxygen," whereas anaerobic activity does not require free oxygen in the body. Cardiovascular exercise, "cardio" for short, is aerobic exercise and includes a wide variety of activities like walking, running, cycling, swimming, rowing, and dancing. These aerobic activities increase your heart rate and the oxygen flow to your cells. They also involve repeatedly moving large muscles—like those in your arms and legs.

Some of the main benefits of cardiovascular activities include strengthening the heart and muscles; preventing cardiovascular disease; boosting mood through the release of endorphins; improving sleep; reducing stress; and healthy weight management. No matter what your fitness level or goals, including some cardiovascular exercise into your routine can improve your overall health and longevity.

During low-intensity, long-duration aerobic activities, the primary fuel source for our bodies is fat. In fact, during periods of rest and daily activities such as light walking, cleaning, and sleeping, fats (both dietary as well as stored) account for 80 to 90 percent of supplied energy. For this reason, while in a state of metabolic ketosis, we are easily able to supply our bodies with the necessary fuel for basic daily function without the need for carbohydrates. This is also why intermittent fasting during exercise or movement can augment progress while on a ketogenic diet (see sidebar on page 13).

This also means that lower-intensity cardio workouts such as walking, jogging, swimming, and cycling are easily supported by a diet very low in carbohydrates. During these activities, the body dips into fat stores to fuel workouts, making them ideal for a keto-fit approach. Many athletes also find that their endurance and the quality of their workouts improve while in a state of metabolic ketosis. This is because the energy stores from fat far outlast those from glucose, making for sustained energy, lack of brain fatigue, and increased stamina from an absence of sugar/glucose crashes. The added bonus of increased body fat burn makes including cardio routines in your keto lifestyle a great fit. Chapter 3 includes a full weight loss–centric meal plan should that be a good match for your goals.

Although cardio does favor fat for fuel, if you are new to a ketogenic or low-carbohydrate way of eating, it may take time for your body to transition to workouts without carbs on board or while in a fasted state. This is completely normal; adapting to any nutrition change takes time. At first, you may not be able to work out for as long as you were previously able to, and you may not be able to keep up your normal paces. Don't beat yourself up. Know that you are working toward a major metabolic transition and be patient with the process. I encourage my clients to focus on nutrition during this phase rather than performance. Sticking to the plan will help your body transition faster; usually within one to four weeks for most. After that period of transition is over, you should quickly be able to work back up to your previous pace and duration.

STRENGTH

As we age, we naturally lose lean body mass (muscle) and gain fat mass, which in turn slows our metabolic rate and can cause other health concerns. In order to overcome (or at least slow) this natural progression, I encourage all my clients—regardless of age or physical fitness goals—to engage in some form of strength activity on a regular basis. Strength training activities typically involve free weights, weight machines, or bodyweight resistance exercises. Not only does strength training help you retain and build lean body mass, but also it helps with bone density and can support healthy weight maintenance, since building muscle is the best way to increase metabolism.

Strength training is an anaerobic activity, meaning it is done without the presence of free oxygen. Anaerobic activities need glucose to produce energy, either in the form of dietary carbohydrates, stored glycogen, or glucose from the breakdown of proteins and fats (gluconeogenesis). In addition to classic strength training workouts, other burst activities like short sprints, hill climbs, high intensity interval training (HIIT exercises), intense core training, and Pilates are also anaerobic activities.

Since anaerobic activities require some glucose for energy, many people transitioning to a ketogenic diet, which is very low in carbohydrates, find that they don't initially feel as strong when performing anaerobic activities. Early in the transition to keto, you may fatigue more quickly or need longer periods of recovery between strength days.

Given this necessary transition time, it is important to assess what your long-term goals are. If improving body composition and endurance are goals for your keto-fit lifestyle, I suggest maintaining ketogenic ratios in meals but reducing weight and reps while including more cardio days during your initial one to three months of going keto.

However, if you have more short-term fitness goals such as an upcoming competition or a desire to lift maximum weight, you will need to supplement with some quick-acting glucose fuel prior to anaerobic strength-based activities. I suggest a small piece of fruit (an apple or banana), a piece of toast, a small bowl of oatmeal, or 8 ounces of chocolate milk to supply your body with the glucose necessary to complete 30 to 60 minutes of anaerobic activity. For longer or more intense workouts, you may need to increase these quantities. At the end of the day, carbs are just a quick form of energy, so if you use them soon after consuming them, like during an anerobic workout, they are processed by your body, not stored, and you can return to a ketogenic lifestyle following the workout. See more on this in the meal plan for building muscle (page 37).

During anaerobic activity, lactic acid is produced as a by-product of the metabolic process and can cause sore muscles if it is not cleared. I recommend engaging in light stretching exercises both before and after anaerobic exercises to allow for proper lactic acid removal, which prevents injury and soreness.

STRETCHING AND REST

Some activities, like stretching or light yoga, do not elevate your heart rate the way cardio and strength training exercises do but still engage important muscle groups. These activities do not rely on glucose and can be done while following a low-carbohydrate ketogenic diet or during fasting.

It is important to incorporate rest days into your fitness routine since this time allows your muscles to recover, adapt, and grow stronger from the work you've put in and prevents injury and fatigue. I recommend at least one rest day each week. This can be a day off completely from your fitness routine while keeping your nutrition plan strong, or it can include light walking, stretching, or light yoga exercises if you prefer.

To Fast or Not to Fast

Intermittent fasting, or time-restricted eating, can deepen your level of ketosis and aid with weight loss or body composition change because it requires your body to rely on stored body fat for energy rather than getting fat from meals or snacks. This increases brain-boosting ketone production and leads to muscle-sparing weight loss. Exercise during the fasting time can really enhance this process. The best activities to include while fasting are aerobic, like cardio and stretching, since they do not rely on much glucose for energy.

The goal of shortening the "window of eating" is not to decrease overall caloric intake, although this may happen naturally, but simply to shorten the time frame in which you ingest those calories. Implementing intermittent fasting should be a gradual progression and never forced. After the first three weeks of a ketogenic diet, you may naturally feel less hunger and transition comfortably to a longer fasting window.

If you wish to transition to intermittent fasting, try pushing breakfast back 30 minutes every two or three days. After a few weeks, you will have gradually increased the time between dinner and breakfast to 16 to 18 hours (for example, dinner at 6:00 p.m. and breakfast at 10:00 a.m.), giving your body more time to burn stored energy.

For many, a schedule with a 6-hour eating window and an 18-hour fasting window means only two meals each day. Others prefer to stick with three meals within that eating window. Do what is comfortable for you. It is important to maintain adequate protein intake, so I do not advise eating only one meal a day for long periods of time. I've designed the meal plans in chapter 3 to include many snack-type breakfast options. To support longer fasting periods, you may prefer to move these breakfasts to become a snack between the first and third meal of the day.

7 Keto-Fit Golden Rules

Changing the way you eat and the way you fuel your workouts can feel overwhelming at first. Aside from following the meal plans and using the recipes in this book, there are a few basic tenets to remember when the going gets tough.

STAY HYDRATED! Within the first few days of starting a ketogenic diet, your body will get rid of stored water as it breaks down stored glycogen. This can lead to dehydration from a loss of electrolytes along with the water. As a general rule, I suggest drinking half of your body weight in ounces daily. So, if you weigh 200 pounds, aim for about 100 ounces of water a day. This can come in the form of unsweetened teas and seltzers, fruit-infused waters, or plain old tap water.

ATTACK CRAVINGS AND DIPS IN ENERGY WITH FAT. If you have a craving for something carb-heavy or feel like you need a quick energy boost after a long workout, attack it with a fatty snack, such as those listed in chapter 8. You are retraining your cells and brain to see fat as a primary fuel source rather than glucose from carbs. By eating fat when cravings hit, you are reinforcing this process and encouraging your body to make the transition.

INCLUDE REST DAYS. No one can do it all, all the time, including you. Be kind to your body, and give it what it needs to be successful. This includes adequate sleep, rest days, and lower-intensity workouts. As your body adjusts from being 100 percent glucose-burning to being ketogenic and fat adapted, you may need to cut back on the intensity or duration of your current physical activity routine until your body embraces the process.

DON'T GO HUNGRY. Even if a goal is weight loss or body composition change, a ketogenic diet does not rely on caloric restriction for success. Hunger will lessen as your body becomes fat adapted, but in the first few weeks, don't worry about how many fat-forward snacks you may need to include during the day to feel energized and keep cravings at bay.

EAT REAL FOOD, AND DON'T FOCUS ON NET CARBS. In an ideal diet, the vast majority of carbohydrates comes from real foods, such as non-starchy vegetables, which contain fiber in addition to a host of essential vitamins and minerals. Avoid packaged "keto-friendly" products that tout low "net carbs," such as breads, cereals, bars, and cookies. Instead, explore the delicious, real food recipes in the chapters that follow. Your body will feel and function better, and many of those processed foods won't even taste so good anymore!

AVOID "CHEAT DAYS," BUT INDULGING HERE AND THERE IS OKAY. You can take your keto-fit lifestyle to the party or restaurant, but I encourage you not to give in to the desire for an all-out "cheat day," which can quickly spiral out of control. Remember carbs are just a form of quick energy, so if you overdo it, include a fasted workout the next morning, focusing on strength training or HIIT activity to burn down any remaining glucose.

KEEP ALCOHOL IN MODERATION. Although many wines and spirits are low in carbohydrates, the body prioritizes processing alcohol over any other energy source, including fat. The liver is the organ responsible for converting fatty acids to ketones for energy. If it is busy detoxifying, it won't be very effective at making ketones. Aside from the metabolic downsides of excessive alcohol consumption, alcohol is dehydrating and inflammatory and can deter progress toward your fitness goals.

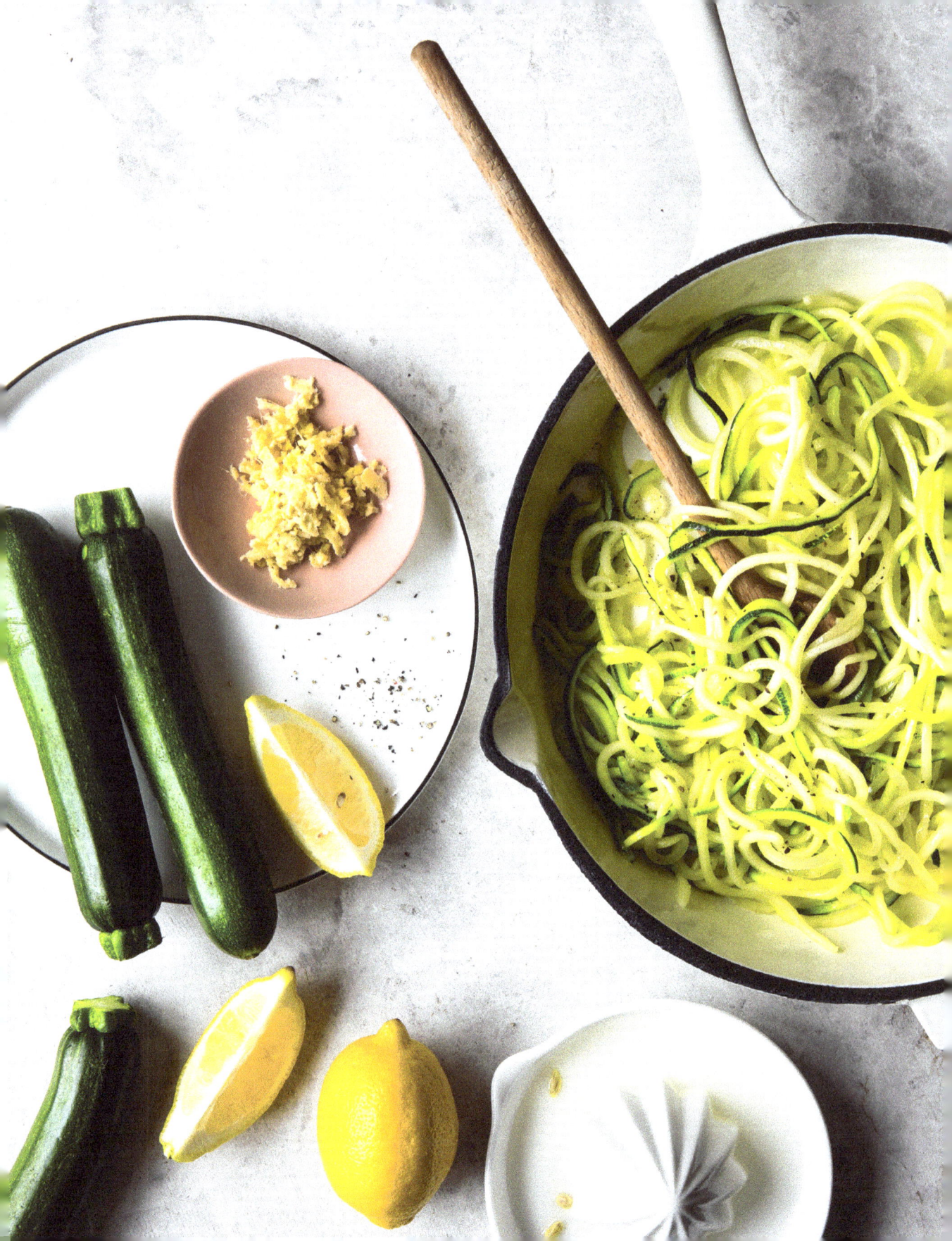

CHAPTER 2

Inside the Keto-Fit Kitchen

NOW IT'S TIME to put all the principles of a keto-fit lifestyle into practice. This chapter will cover everything you'll need, from staple ingredients to kitchen essentials, to kick-start your journey toward optimal fitness through a ketogenic dietary approach.

Beginning Your Keto Fitness Journey

Like so many things in life, good nutrition is all about planning ahead. Knowing which foods are best for a sustainable ketogenic diet that fuels your activity—and also understanding how they fit together as complete, macronutrient-balanced meals—is key to success. No matter how determined you may be, if you are overly hungry and without supplies or a plan, making the best decision for your nutrition becomes difficult. Have no fear; in this chapter, I will help you get prepared by cleansing your kitchen of the foods that will prevent success while stocking up on the foods and items that will make delicious meal prep a breeze.

The Keto Kitchen Cleanse

In order to achieve and maintain nutritional ketosis, the amount of carbohydrates at each meal must be kept exceptionally low, which means excluding foods that derive the majority of their energy (calories) from carbohydrates.

The obvious offenders are sweets, breads, pastas, and cereals, but even healthy foods such as fruits, starchy vegetables, and whole grains contain levels of carbohydrate too high to be included in most ketogenic meal plans. Keeping these around can derail even the best intentions, so it's easier if they are out of sight and out of mind. Foods to avoid keeping in your keto kitchen include:

- Beans and legumes
- Beer and hard cider
- Cereals and granolas
- Cookies and candies
- Crackers, pretzels, and chips (even gluten-free versions)
- Dried fruit like raisins
- Fruit spreads, including jams, jellies, and preserves
- Grains like rice, pasta, and quinoa
- High-sugar fruits like bananas, pineapples, and mangos
- Low-fat or skim milks and cheeses
- Regular ketchup, barbecue sauce, and other condiments containing sugar
- Seasoning blends that include sugar, like cinnamon-sugar blends
- Sugar, brown sugar, honey, maple syrup, agave, and corn syrup
- Sugary beverages like fruit juices and soda (including diet soda)

- Sweetened coffee creamers
- Sweetened teas and coffee drinks
- Sweetened yogurts
- White and whole-wheat flours, chickpea flour, and rice flour

Keto Kitchen Essentials

A well-stocked kitchen makes meal prep and balanced eating so much easier. Although some of these kitchen essentials may require an initial outlay of cash, having these ingredients, supplements, and equipment on hand will not only save you time but also money in the long run.

FRIDGE AND FREEZER STAPLES

Fresh and frozen ingredients will serve as the backbone for the recipes in this book.

EGGS are a complete protein source and will last in the refrigerator for up to two weeks. Free-range eggs offer the best-quality omega-3 fats and are thus well worth the extra expense.

FRESH VEGETABLES such as cucumber, bell pepper, cherry tomatoes, celery, broccoli, cauliflower, radishes, and carrots are filled with micronutrients (think vitamins and minerals). These are the best source of carbohydrates on your keto-fit nutrition plan.

FROZEN BERRIES such as strawberries, blueberries, raspberries, and blackberries are anti-inflammatory powerhouses that are delicious in smoothies, yogurt bowls, and baked keto-friendly goods.

FROZEN MEATS, FISH, AND POULTRY are good to keep on hand for last-minute meals. Also, buying proteins in bulk and freezing individual portions is a cost-effective way to include quality protein sources in your keto-fit lifestyle.

FROZEN VEGETABLES are just as healthy as their fresh counterparts and are much easier to store. Consider stocking your freezer with vegetables like broccoli, spinach, asparagus, Brussels sprouts, bell peppers, cauliflower, riced cauliflower, zucchini, and yellow squash. Avoid vegetable blends containing peas, corn, beans, and potatoes.

GRASS-FED BUTTER is a versatile source of quality, anti-inflammatory fat.

MAYONNAISE is a perfect base for tasty sauces and dressings that can help increase the fat ratios in your meals. I love avocado- or olive oil–based mayos for their anti-inflammatory fats and rich flavor.

NUTS AND SEEDS such as almonds, walnuts, pecans, macadamias, hazelnuts, Brazil nuts, pistachios, flaxseed, chia seeds, pumpkin seeds, and sesame seeds (store in the freezer to stay fresh longer!) are a convenient and portable heart-healthy fat that add a great dose of fiber and protein for on-the-go nutrition.

QUALITY CHEESES such as parmesan, cheddar, mozzarella, feta, goat cheese, and plain full-fat cream cheese add flavorful fat and protein to a wide variety of dishes.

SALAD GREENS such as arugula, spinach, kale, baby lettuces, and romaine provide important minerals and vitamins and are a great base for delicious keto salads and entrées.

WHOLE-MILK GREEK YOGURT AND FULL-FAT COTTAGE CHEESE are inexpensive and convenient sources of post-workout protein.

PANTRY STAPLES

The recipes in this book will lean heavily on a small number of pantry items, some that you may already have and others that you'll need to purchase.

ALMOND AND COCONUT FLOURS are great for keto-friendly baked goods and treats.

AVOCADOS, a keto favorite because they provide tons of heart-healthy fats, are considered a pantry item because you should store unripe avocados in a dark place at room temperature. Once they start to ripen, move them to the refrigerator so that they last longer.

BROTH OR STOCK (chicken, beef, and vegetable) is nice to have on hand for homemade soups and stews.

CANNED DICED TOMATOES, PUREED TOMATOES, AND TOMATO PASTE with no sugar added are a nice pantry option for when fresh tomatoes aren't in season and on hand. Canned tomatoes help add great flavor to simple dishes that come together on the fly.

CANNED SEAFOOD, such as tuna packed in oil, is an easy, convenient, and portable protein option on the go.

OILS will be your main cooking fats. Olive oil, avocado oil, coconut oil, and sesame oil provide heart-healthy and delicious fats for easy meals.

SPICES AND DRIED HERBS such as cinnamon, ground ginger, garlic powder, chili powder, ground cumin, red pepper flakes, dill, rosemary, parsley, and thyme bring flavor and variety to dishes to prevent the "same ol' chicken" syndrome.

SUGAR-FREE SWEETENERS, such as monk fruit, stevia, or Swerve (optional), make for keto-friendly baked goods and treats.

UNSWEETENED NUT AND SEED BUTTERS, such as almond, sunflower, and tahini (sesame seed paste), are healthy snacks as well as bases for dressings and sauces.

VINEGARS, like red- and white-wine vinegars, unseasoned rice vinegar, and balsamic vinegar, are staples for homemade dressings and marinades and for seasoning meats and vegetables.

VITAMINS AND SUPPLEMENTS

Although nutrient-dense foods are the best source of energy and dietary medicine, there are a few supplements that I recommend.

CURCUMIN (an active component of turmeric) is frequently used to reduce joint pain and can help with recovery from intense exercise. Turmeric, the main component of many curry powders and fragrant spice blends, is delicious in cooking, but the amount needed for therapeutic benefits greatly exceeds what we are able to ingest from meals alone.

ELECTROLYTES (sodium, potassium, calcium, and magnesium) are present in dietary sources like avocados, chicken or beef broth, and fatty fish such as salmon and mackerel. Try an over-the-counter magnesium supplement if muscle soreness, constipation, headache, or other signs of dehydration persist. Sports drinks without added sugars are good options for excessively sweaty workouts or during early stages of a ketogenic diet to prevent "keto flu."

FISH OIL (OMEGA-3) includes the essential omega-3 fatty acids eicosapentaenoic acid (EPA) and docosahexaenoic acid (DHA). Fatty fish such as wild-caught salmon, mackerel, sardines, and anchovies are excellent sources of these anti-inflammatory powerhouses. If you are unable to include adequate food sources (three or four servings per week) of EPA and DHA in your diet, take a fish oil or omega-3 supplement that includes both EPA and DHA.

MCT (MEDIUM-CHAIN TRIGLYCERIDE) OIL is absorbed differently in our digestive tract due to the unique length of this fatty acid, allowing for immediate conversion to ketones. The rapid increase in ketone levels helps with energy, mental clarity, and satiety.

TART CHERRY CAPSULES are a good option for reaping all the health benefits of cherries without consuming the high amounts of natural sugars that the fruits contain. Dark cherries have powerful antioxidant properties and aid in recovery in athletes.

EQUIPMENT ESSENTIALS

You don't have to be a professional chef or have a state-of-the-art kitchen to prepare ketogenic meals, but having the following tools will make it all come together faster.

BAKING SHEETS don't need to be fancy to work. They can be lined with aluminum foil or parchment paper before using to minimize cleanup time.

A BOX GRATER, ZESTER, OR MICROPLANE is the best way to create fresh flavor and added nutrition from citrus zest, grated cheese, and even shredded vegetables.

A FOOD PROCESSOR will bring monetary and time savings by helping you make homemade riced cauliflower, finely slivered or chopped vegetables, pesto, dressings, sauces, and nut butters.

A GARLIC PRESS will help impart great garlic flavor into sauces, dips, and dressings without the harshness from larger garlic pieces.

GLASS BAKING DISHES, including 9-by-13-inch and 8-by-8-inch dishes, are used in many of the recipes in this book and can double as storage for leftovers as well.

GLASS OR PLASTIC STORAGE CONTAINERS in various sizes are a worthwhile investment, since the meal plans in the following chapters save you a lot of kitchen time by having you cook ahead and store leftovers. In a pinch, freezer-friendly zip-top plastic bags will work for cooked proteins and soups.

AN IMMERSION BLENDER is great for making smoothies, dressings, sauces, and soups. Immersion blenders are affordable, versatile, and easy to clean.

MEASURING CUPS AND SPOONS, ranging from ¼ cup to 1 cup and from ⅛ teaspoon to 1 tablespoon, are necessary for accurately measuring recipe ingredients.

SAUCEPANS AND SKILLETS in a variety of sizes will come in handy. If you are doubling any of the recipes for leftovers or enjoying with friends and family, you will want to have larger pots and pans for cooking. I love a 10- to 12-inch cast-iron skillet for searing fish and meats, but a regular medium skillet will be just fine.

SHARP KNIVES are the most important tool for any chef. Quality, sharp knives can help prevent kitchen accidents and make meal prep a breeze.

A SPIRALIZER at home allows you to make spiralized veggies—like the ones many grocery stores offer in the refrigerated produce section.

A MEDIUM WHISK allows you to make sauces smooth and eggs fluffy.

Shopping for Affordable Keto Ingredients

Following a heathy keto-fit lifestyle does not have to mean high grocery bills and a house full of expensive ingredients. There are several tricks to staying keto while keeping costs minimal and within weekly budgets.

Buy in bulk. Many proteins, such as meats, poultry, and seafood, can be bought in bulk at a cheaper cost per pound and frozen in individual portions. You can also cook larger cuts, portion them, and freeze them for easy ready-to-go meals throughout the week.

Use frozen vegetables. It is a myth that frozen vegetables are less nutritious than their fresh counterparts. Buying frozen vegetables, such as chopped spinach, broccoli, and cauliflower, cuts costs and saves trips to the grocery store.

Buy what's in season. If fresh is what you crave, buying vegetables and berries when they are in season will save you money and provide the best-tasting meals and snacks.

Ditch the name brand. Many store-brand or off-label options for pricey ingredients such as almond flour, nuts, seeds, oils, and nut butters are of equal quality to the name brands. Be sure to read labels and compare ingredients and be on the lookout for additives such as sugars or processed oils like canola or palm oil.

Stick to the list. Make a grocery list before going to the store (and never arrive hungry!) to avoid having last-minute items pop into your cart.

Tips for Meal Prepping

If you're not a fan of spending hours in the kitchen to prepare home-cooked meals, there are many ways to save time for the things in life you really enjoy (like an extra-long run or swim on a sunny day). Although the recipes that follow are designed to be quick and easy and the meal plans in chapter 3 all give great tips for time-saving prep, here are a couple of ways to get food on the table even faster and avoid hungry temptations.

COOK ONCE; ENJOY MANY TIMES. Not everyone loves leftovers, but repurposing certain components of a dish for a variety of uses can be a huge time-saver and cuts down on frequent cooking. For example, try making the Spinach Shakshuka (page 55) for a weekend brunch and then serving the leftovers midweek for a light dinner. No need for extra prep!

PREP AHEAD. Picking a day of the week to prep staples like chopped onions and fresh herbs, cut vegetables, or batch-grill or bake proteins such as meat or chicken can save you significant time getting meals on the table during the week. And the best part is, by doing it all at once, you cut down on cleanup time.

BATCH RECIPES. If you double one or two recipes every week and freeze the leftovers in single-serve portions, over time you will have built up the healthiest array of ready-to-go frozen entrées at your fingertips. These can be lifesavers for last-minute meals.

DON'T ARRIVE AT A RESTAURANT OR PARTY HUNGRY! It can be hard to resist the chips, breads, and other carb-heavy fillers if you haven't eaten all day. One or two hours before dining out, enjoy a snack with healthy fats, such as Coconut–Nut Butter Power Balls (page 98) or some Cashew Hummus (page 103) with celery to help keep a handle on hunger and cravings.

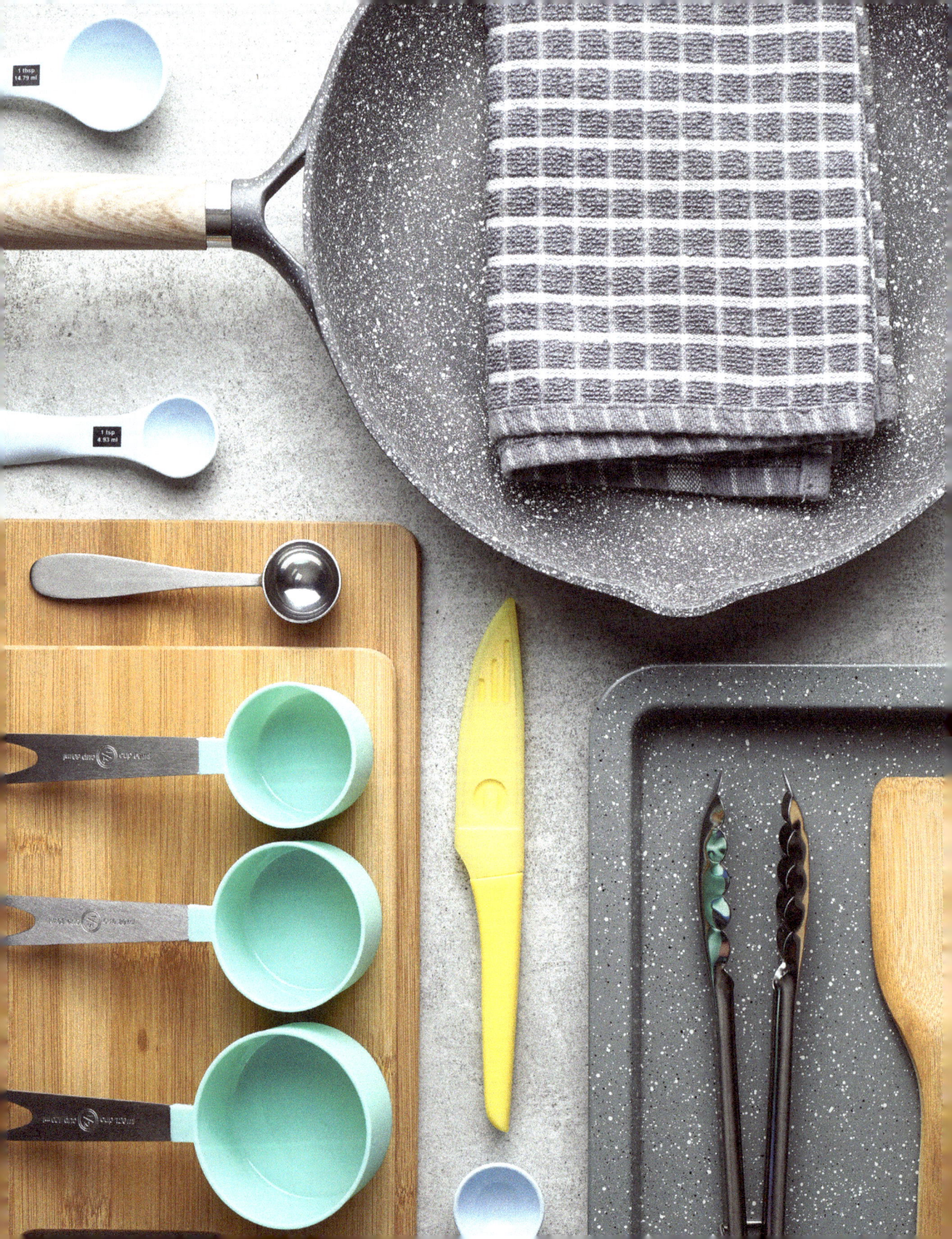

CHAPTER 3

Keto-Fit Meal Plans

SUCCESSFULLY ADAPTING THE KETO-FIT LIFESTYLE into your routine begins with a solid plan. The following four one-week plans provide the perfect framework and are catered to specific fitness needs. Each plan is designed for one person, although many recipes make leftovers that can be frozen for later (see the storage tips at the end of each recipe); scale up the quantity and double-check the serving sizes on the recipes if you are feeding more than one. You'll find a shopping list and a meal prep schedule to make a full week of home-cooked keto goodness with minimal effort. The first prep day covers meals for the first half of the week, and another midweek prep day will see you through the rest. By following these guides, you will be able to shop once, prep twice, and eat all week long.

Making Adjustments

If a dietary plan is going to find any success, it needs to fit your lifestyle and preferences. Making adjustments to the plans and recipes that follow, whether out of personal preference or dietary restrictions, is 100 percent a part of the keto-fit lifestyle. Feel free to switch out proteins, such as chicken or seafood for pork or beef, but keep portion sizes consistent to keep keto ratios optimal for success. I encourage all my clients with body composition or weight-loss goals to give their bodies the opportunity to use stored body fat for fuel rather than always relying on dietary intake. For this reason, the weekends in the following plans include a "brunch" along with a heavier snack option to assist you in slowly transitioning to longer periods of fasting. However, you can stick to the breakfast, lunch, and dinner schedule over the weekend if you prefer, using the convenience breakfast options found in the plan or other recipes in this book.

Post-workout snack options are included in each plan, but prioritize balanced, satiating meals over snacks; you can adjust your eating schedule accordingly. For example, if you favor morning workouts, aim to have your breakfast 30 to 90 minutes following that workout, negating the need for a snack. Similarly, if you prefer midday or evening workouts, aim to have lunch or dinner 30 to 90 minutes following that exercise, and you may not need snacks throughout the day. It is important to note that the snacks in the meal plans are optional and should be consumed as needed.

What to Do If You Fall Off the Keto Wagon

Change is hard. If you have a bad day or feel you have "fallen off the wagon," put it behind you and get right back to your plan. One incident will not derail you from long-term success. What hinders long-term success is the snowball effect that is inevitable when we have an "all or nothing" mentality. Remember that no one is perfect and that some days will be better and easier than others; just don't let the hard days take over. You got this!

Here are some tips I give my clients when they feel they need a reset:

- ▶ Practice intermittent fasting for 16 to 24 hours to help burn off excess glucose from overindulgence in carbohydrates.

- ▶ Engage in fasted strength training, HIIT activities, or both to work through glucose and stored glycogen.

- ▶ Attack carb and sugar cravings with fats. Fill up on keto goodness, and do not skimp on calories or quantities. To fully reset your body and brain, it can't feel deprived.

Keto Jump Start

The goal of this weeklong meal plan is to help your body transition into ketosis, becoming acclimated to the keto-fit lifestyle while controlling cravings, maintaining steady energy stores, avoiding symptoms of the dreaded "keto flu," and enjoying tasty yet easy-to-prepare meals.

Although you may have to adjust your current workout routine while your body adapts to ketosis (see page 9), you should have no problem continuing low-intensity cardio activity such as walking, jogging, swimming, cycling, and stretching.

MEAL PLAN

	BREAKFAST	LUNCH	DINNER	SNACK
MON	Broccoli and Cheddar Mini Quiches (page 50) (2)	Guacamole Salad (page 64) with 2 ounces canned tuna	Slow Cooker Chicken Tikka Masala (page 75) over 2 cups baby spinach leaves	Chocolate-Peanut Butter Cups (page 111)
TUES	Leftover Broccoli and Cheddar Mini Quiches (2)	Leftover Guacamole Salad with 2 ounces canned tuna	Leftover Slow Cooker Chicken Tikka Masala over riced cauliflower	Leftover Chocolate-Peanut Butter Cups
WED	½ cup plain Greek yogurt mixed with 2 tablespoons heavy cream, ¼ cup berries, 2 tablespoons flaxseed (or nuts)	Leftover Slow Cooker Chicken Tikka Masala over 2 cups baby spinach leaves	Thai-Inspired Ground Pork Lettuce Cups (page 85)	Leftover Chocolate-Peanut Butter Cups
THURS	Leftover Broccoli and Cheddar Mini Quiches (2)	Leftover Slow Cooker Chicken Tikka Masala over 2 cups baby spinach leaves	Flank Steak with Easy Chimichurri Sauce (page 92) over 2 cups baby spinach leaves	Celery sticks with 2 tablespoons Cashew Hummus (page 103)

	BREAKFAST	LUNCH	DINNER	SNACK
FRI	½ cup plain Greek yogurt mixed with 2 tablespoons heavy cream, ¼ cup berries, 2 tablespoons flaxseed (or nuts)	Leftover Flank Steak with Easy Chimichurri over 2 cups baby spinach leaves	Leftover Thai-Inspired Ground Pork Lettuce Cups	Celery sticks with 2 tablespoons Cashew Hummus
SAT	Skip breakfast today and enjoy a larger post-workout snack	Leftover Thai-Inspired Ground Pork Lettuce Cups	Leftover Flank Steak with Easy Chimichurri Sauce over riced cauliflower	2 tablespoons Cashew Hummus on a 90-Second Keto Dinner Roll (page 99)
SUN	Skip breakfast today and enjoy a larger brunch or lunch	Leftover Flank Steak with Easy Chimichurri Sauce served as a sandwich with a 90-Second Keto Dinner Roll (page 99)	Leftover Thai-Inspired Ground Pork Lettuce Cups served with riced cauliflower	2 tablespoons Cashew Hummus with celery sticks

Keto-Fit Meal Plans ◂ 31

SHOPPING LIST

PRODUCE
Avocados (4)
Blueberries (1 [6-ounce] container, or 6 ounces frozen)
Celery (1 bunch)
Cilantro (1 large or 2 small bunches)
Garlic (2 heads)
Ginger (1 [4-inch] piece)
Lemons (2)
Lettuce, Bibb (1 head)
Lime (1)
Onion, yellow (1)
Orange (1)
Scallions (1 bunch)
Spinach, baby (16 ounces)
Tomatoes, cherry (1 pint)

DAIRY AND EGGS
Butter, unsalted (8 ounces)
Cheese, cheddar, shredded (1 [6-ounce] bag)
Eggs, large (14)
Greek yogurt, whole-milk, plain (8 ounces)
Heavy cream (½ pint)

MEAT AND SEAFOOD
Chicken, thighs, boneless, skinless (2 pounds)
Beef, flank steak (1 pound)
Pork, sausage, mild, ground (1 pound)

FROZEN
Broccoli (1 [10-ounce] bag)
Cauliflower, riced (1 [10-ounce] bag)

HERBS AND SPICES
Curry powder
Garlic powder
Onion powder
Peppercorns, black
Salt, kosher

PANTRY
Baking powder
Cashews, raw
Chocolate chips, sugar-free
Cocoa powder, unsweetened
Coconut milk, full-fat, unsweetened (2 [13½-ounce] cans)
Fish sauce
Flaxseed
Flour, almond
Oil, coconut, refined
Oil, olive, extra-virgin
Oil, sesame, toasted
Peanut butter, creamy, unsweetened
Tahini
Tamari
Tomato paste, no-sugar-added (1 [4½-ounce] tube)
Tuna (1 [4-ounce] can)

PREP DAY #1
Estimated prep time: 1 hour 20 minutes, plus 4 to 5 hours inactive time

1. Preheat the oven to 350°F and prep your kitchen.
2. Make the Broccoli and Cheddar Mini Quiches.
3. While the mini quiches are in the oven, make the Chocolate–Peanut Butter Cups. Store in an airtight container in the freezer.
4. Prep the dressing for the Guacamole Salad (follow step 2 in the recipe). Divide the dressing into 4 airtight containers and store in the refrigerator.
5. Chop the tomatoes, scallion, and cilantro for the Guacamole Salad. Put them together in an airtight container. Don't add the avocados or dressing until just before serving.
6. Prepare the Slow Cooker Chicken Tikka Masala and cook in the slow cooker for 4 to 6 hours.
7. Once the mini quiches and chicken tikka masala are cool, pack into individual airtight containers.

PREP DAY #2
Estimated prep time: 20 minutes, plus 8 hours overnight to soak

1. Soak the cashews overnight for the Cashew Hummus.
2. Make the pork mixture for the Thai-Inspired Ground Pork Lettuce Cups by following steps 1 to 5 in the recipe. Allow to cool, then store in airtight containers in the refrigerator.
3. Make the chimichurri sauce for the Flank Steak with Easy Chimichurri (step 3), cover, and store in the refrigerator. Because the steak grills so quickly, wait to cook the steak until just before serving.

Weight Loss

To support weight-loss goals on the keto-fit journey, this plan keeps macros ideal for a fat-burning, ketogenic metabolic state. This plan emphasizes meals rather than snacks, encouraging your body to rely on fat storage for energy between meals. If you have cravings or need snacks during the first half of the week, that is absolutely fine. Just be sure to avoid snacking out of habit; don't snack if you don't feel hunger between meals.

As you plan your exercise for the week, remember that a blend of cardio for fat burn and light strength training for lean body mass preservation and metabolic boost is ideal for weight-loss goals.

MEAL PLAN

	BREAKFAST	LUNCH	DINNER	SNACK
MON	Fully-Fueled Protein Shake (page 51)	Fuel Up Arugula Salad (page 60) with 2 ounces canned tuna	Pesto Steak and Broccoli Foil Packs (page 91)	1 hard-boiled egg
TUES	Fully-Fueled Protein Shake (page 51)	Leftover Fuel Up Arugula Salad with 1 hard-boiled egg	Leftover Pesto Steak and Broccoli Foil Packs	2 tablespoons almonds or walnuts
WED	2 eggs scrambled in 1 tablespoon olive oil topped with ½ sliced avocado	Leftover Fuel Up Arugula Salad with 2 ounces canned tuna	Greek Stuffed Chicken Breasts (page 79) with side salad and 2 tablespoons Crave-Worthy Caesar Dressing (page 102)	1 tablespoon peanut butter with celery sticks
THURS	Fully-Fueled Protein Shake (page 51)	Leftover Pesto Steak and Broccoli Foil Packs	Peanut and Lime Zoodles (page 67) topped with 1 fried egg	1 hard-boiled egg

	BREAKFAST	LUNCH	DINNER	SNACK
FRI	2 eggs scrambled in 1 tablespoon olive oil topped with ½ sliced avocado	Leftover Peanut and Lime Zoodles topped with 2 ounces canned tuna	Leftover Greek Stuffed Chicken Breasts with side salad and 2 tablespoons Crave-Worthy Caesar Dressing	1 tablespoon peanut butter with celery sticks
SAT	Skip breakfast today and include a larger post-workout snack	Leftover Peanut and Lime Zoodles topped with 1 fried egg	Chorizo and Cheese-Stuffed Poblanos (page 83)	Cookie Dough Fat Bombs (page 108)
SUN	Skip breakfast and enjoy a larger lunch	Leftover Chorizo and Cheese-Stuffed Poblanos	Leftover Peanut and Lime Zoodles topped with 2 ounces canned tuna	Leftover Cookie Dough Fat Bombs

SHOPPING LIST

PRODUCE
Arugula, baby (10 ounces)
Avocado (1)
Bell pepper, red (1)
Broccoli florets (1 cup or 10 ounces frozen)
Celery (1 bunch)
Garlic (1 head)
Lemons (2)
Limes (2)
Mushrooms, sliced (8 ounces)
Peppers, poblano (4 large)
Salad greens (6 ounces)
Zucchini (2 medium)

DAIRY AND EGGS
Butter, unsalted (8 ounces)
Cheese, feta, crumbled (8 ounces)
Cheese, Mexican blend, shredded (8 ounces)
Cream cheese, full-fat (8 ounces)
Eggs, large (9)

MEAT AND SEAFOOD
Beef, flank steak (1 pound)
Chicken, breasts, boneless, skinless (2; about 1 pound)
Chorizo, ground (8 ounces)

FROZEN
Broccoli (1 [12-ounce] bag)
Spinach (1 [10-ounce] bag)

HERBS AND SPICES
Garlic powder
Ginger, ground
Oregano, dried
Peppercorns, black
Salt, kosher

PANTRY
Almond milk, unsweetened (28 ounces)
Anchovy paste
Basil pesto (1 [4-ounce] jar)
Chocolate chips, mini, sugar-free
Coconut milk, full-fat, unsweetened (2 [13½-ounce] cans)
Collagen peptides or other unsweetened protein powder
Flour, almond
Mayonnaise
Mustard, Dijon
Oil, olive, extra-virgin
Oil, sesame, toasted
Olives, Kalamata
Peanut butter, unsweetened
Sugar-free granulated sweetener, such as Swerve
Tamari
Tuna (2 [4-ounce] cans)
Vanilla extract
Vinegar, balsamic
Walnuts (1¼ cups)
Worcestershire sauce

PREP DAY #1
Estimated prep time: 50 minutes
1. Make the Cookie Dough Fat Bombs. Store in the freezer.
2. Boil 3 eggs. Let cool, then store in the refrigerator.
3. Make the dressing for the Fuel Up Arugula Salad (follow step 1 of the recipe). Store covered in the refrigerator.
4. Prepare the Pesto Steak and Broccoli Foil Packs (steps 2 to 6 from the recipe). Store the prepared packs in the refrigerator until ready to grill. Store any packs that you won't be eating this week in the freezer.

PREP DAY #2
Estimated prep time: 1 hour 45 minutes
1. Prepare and bake the Greek Stuffed Chicken Breasts. Let cool completely before storing covered in the refrigerator. While the chicken bakes, continue the prep.
2. Make the Crave-Worthy Caesar Dressing. Store in an airtight container in the refrigerator.
3. Make the sauce for the Peanut and Lime Zoodles by following step 1 in the recipe. Store the sauce in an airtight container in the refrigerator.
4. Make the vegetables for the Peanut and Lime Zoodles (steps 2 to 5) of the recipe. Let cool and then store in individual containers in the refrigerator. Reheat before tossing with the sauce and raw zoodles to serve.
5. Prepare and stuff the Chorizo and Cheese–Stuffed Poblanos (steps 1 to 10 of the recipe). Store covered in the refrigerator until ready to bake.

Muscle Building

Including more strength training, weight-bearing exercise, and HIIT activities will help build lean body mass and improve body composition when following a ketogenic meal plan. These types of anaerobic exercises require slightly higher amounts of carbohydrates than aerobic cardio activity, and the recipes included in this plan reflect those nutrient needs. Time your meals around exercise, with the goal of eating a meal 30 to 90 minutes after activity. If this is not possible due to your schedule, including a post-workout higher-protein snack will help you recover and replenish following exercise. The pre-workout snack is optional and only suggested if you feel you are lagging in workouts or hungrier between meals.

MEAL PLAN

	BREAKFAST	PRE-WORKOUT	LUNCH	DINNER	POST-WORKOUT
MON	Nutty Baked Oatmeal (page 52)	Half of a 90-Second Keto Dinner Roll (page 99) with 1 tablespoon peanut butter	Easy Greek Salad (page 65) with 4 ounces canned tuna	Herby Orange Baked Chicken (page 71) with Riced Cauliflower and Herb Salad (page 66)	Coconut-Nut Butter Power Balls (page 98)
TUES	Leftover Nutty Baked Oatmeal	1 hard-boiled egg	Leftover Easy Greek Salad with half portion leftover Herby Orange Baked Chicken	Easy Slow-Cooked Ribs (page 84) with leftover Riced Cauliflower and Herb Salad	Leftover Coconut-Nut Butter Power Balls
WED	Leftover Nutty Baked Oatmeal	1 hard-boiled egg	Leftover Easy Greek Salad with half portion leftover Herby Orange Baked Chicken	Leftover Easy Slow-Cooked Ribs with leftover Riced Cauliflower and Herb Salad	Leftover Coconut-Nut Butter Power Balls
THURS	Breakfast Pizza (page 56)	Half serving leftover Nutty Baked Oatmeal	Leftover Easy Slow-Cooked Ribs with leftover Riced Cauliflower and Herb Salad	Leftover Herby Orange Baked Chicken with 2 cups mixed greens and 2 tablespoons Lemon-Tahini Sauce (page 96)	Leftover Coconut-Nut Butter Power Balls

	BREAKFAST	PRE-WORKOUT	LUNCH	DINNER	POST-WORKOUT
FRI	Leftover Breakfast Pizza	Half serving leftover Nutty Baked Oatmeal	Half serving leftover Herby Orange Baked Chicken with 1 tablespoon mayonnaise on 90-Second Keto Dinner Roll (page 99)	Corn Bread Taco Pie (page 82)	Leftover Coconut–Nut Butter Power Balls
SAT	Leftover Breakfast Pizza	Half of a 90-Second Keto Dinner Roll (page 99) with 1 tablespoon peanut butter	Half serving leftover Herby Orange Baked Chicken over 2 cups mixed greens with 2 tablespoons leftover Lemon-Tahini Sauce	Leftover Corn Bread Taco Pie	Leftover Coconut–Nut Butter Power Balls
SUN	Skip breakfast today and enjoy a larger brunch	1 hard-boiled egg	Breakfast Pizza (page 56) and half serving leftover Nutty Baked Oatmeal	Leftover Corn Bread Taco Pie	Leftover Coconut–Nut Butter Power Balls

SHOPPING LIST

PRODUCE
Avocados, ripe, large (2)
Bell pepper, red (1)
Cauliflower (1 small head)
Celery (1 bunch)
Cucumber (1)
Garlic (1 head)
Lemons (4)
Lettuce, romaine (1 head)
Mint (1 bunch)
Mixed salad greens (6 ounces)
Onion, red (1)
Orange, medium (1)
Parsley, Italian (1 bunch)
Tomatoes, roma (4)

DAIRY AND EGGS
Butter, unsalted (8 ounces)
Cheese, feta (4 ounces)
Cheese, Mexican blend, shredded (2 [6-ounce] bags)
Cheese, mozzarella, shredded (2 [6-ounce] bags)
Cream cheese, full-fat (8 ounces)
Eggs, large (18)
Heavy cream (½ pint)
Sour cream (8 ounces)

MEAT AND SEAFOOD
Beef, grass-fed, ground (1 pound)
Chicken, thighs, boneless, skinless (1¼ pounds)
Pepperoni (8 ounces)
Pork, baby back ribs (1 [2½- to 3-pound] rack)

FROZEN
Corn (10 ounces)

HERBS AND SPICES
Cinnamon, ground
Garlic powder
Italian seasoning blend
Oregano, dried
Peppercorns, black
Salt, kosher
Taco seasoning
Thyme, dried

PANTRY
Almond milk, unsweetened (24 ounces)
Baking powder
Chia seeds
Coconut flakes, unsweetened
Collagen peptides
Cornmeal
Flaxseed, ground
Flour, almond
Ketchup, no-sugar-added
Marinara sauce, no-sugar-added (4 ounces)
Mayonnaise
Oats, steel-cut, quick-cooking
Oil, olive, extra-virgin
Olives, Kalamata
Peanut butter, unsweetened
Salsa, no-sugar-added, jarred
Sugar-free sweetener, granulated, such as Swerve
Tahini
Tamari
Tuna (1 [4-ounce] can)
Vanilla extract
Vinegar, apple cider
Walnuts

PREP DAY #1

Estimated prep time: 1 hour 30 minutes, plus 6 hours inactive time

1. Preheat the oven to 375°F and prep your kitchen.
2. Make the Coconut–Nut Butter Power Balls. Store in the freezer.
3. Boil 3 eggs. Let cool and store in the refrigerator.
4. Prepare and bake the Nutty Baked Oatmeal. Once it is cooled, store in individual airtight containers in the refrigerator.
5. While the oatmeal cooks, prep the Easy Greek Salad (follow steps 1 to 3 in the recipe), keeping the salad and dressing separate in the refrigerator.
6. Prepare and cook the Easy Slow-Cooked Ribs without finishing (follow only steps 1 to 3).
7. Prep the cauliflower, herbs, and vegetables for the Riced Cauliflower and Herb Salad per steps 1 to 3. Make the dressing and store in separate containers in the refrigerator until ready to serve.

PREP DAY #2

Estimated prep time: 55 minutes

1. Preheat the oven to 375°F.
2. Make the Lemon-Tahini Sauce. Cover and store in the refrigerator.
3. Make the filling for the Corn Bread Taco Pie (follow steps 2 to 4 of the recipe). Store covered in the refrigerator until ready to bake.
4. Prepare the Breakfast Pizza completely. Cool and store in the refrigerator.

Maintaining

Now that you have seen success with your keto-fit nutrition plan and become keto adapted, maintaining progress in health, nutrition, and fitness goals is easy! I suggest sticking with three meals daily and only using the post-workout snack options when schedules do not allow for a meal 30 to 90 minutes following exercise or when workouts are longer and more intense. Engaging in fasted cardio or light strength training activities can help maintain a state of ketosis as well as compensate for higher-carb days. If you feel increased carb or sugar cravings or greater hunger between meals, increase fat servings at each meal before resorting to between-meal snacks. For example, add extra olive oil or dressing to your salad or try some of Molly's Flavor-Filled Mayo (page 97) with your grilled meats, fish, or vegetables for a delicious way to keep fat ratios ideal for long-term success.

MEAL PLAN

	BREAKFAST	LUNCH	DINNER	POST-WORKOUT
MON	Overnight Smoothie Bowl (page 54) (without berries)	Fuel Up Arugula Salad (page 60) with 2 ounces canned tuna	Baked Chicken Alfredo with Spinach (page 78)	Coconut–Nut Butter Power Balls (page 98)
TUES	2 eggs scrambled in 1 tablespoon olive oil topped with ½ sliced avocado	Leftover Fuel Up Arugula Salad with 2 ounces canned tuna	Leftover Baked Chicken Alfredo with Spinach	Leftover Coconut-Nut Butter Power Balls
WED	Overnight Smoothie Bowl (page 54) (without berries)	Leftover Fuel Up Arugula Salad with 2 ounces canned tuna	Simple Ceviche Salad (page 77)	Leftover Coconut-Nut Butter Power Balls
THURS	½ cup plain Greek yogurt mixed with 2 tablespoons heavy cream, ¼ cup berries, 2 tablespoons flaxseed (or nuts)	Leftover Simple Ceviche Salad	Leftover Baked Chicken Alfredo with Spinach	Leftover Coconut-Nut Butter Power Balls

	BREAKFAST	LUNCH	DINNER	POST-WORKOUT
FRI	Fully-Fueled Protein Shake (page 51)	2 ounces tuna and 2 tablespoons mayonnaise on a 90-Second Keto Dinner Roll (page 99)	Leftover Simple Ceviche Salad	Leftover Coconut–Nut Butter Power Balls
SAT	2-egg omelet with 1 ounce cream cheese and ¼ cup spinach and mushrooms cooked in 1 tablespoon butter	Leftover Simple Ceviche Salad	Braised Beef Short Ribs (page 93) with 2 cups mixed greens with Creamy Avocado Dressing (page 101)	Leftover Coconut–Nut Butter Power Balls
SUN	Skip breakfast today and enjoy a larger brunch	2-egg omelet with 1 ounce cream cheese and ¼ cup spinach and mushrooms cooked in 1 tablespoon butter and topped with ½ avocado	Leftover Braised Beef Short Ribs with 2 cups mixed greens with leftover Creamy Avocado Dressing	Leftover Coconut–Nut Butter Power Balls

SHOPPING LIST

PRODUCE
Avocados (5)
Arugula, baby (10 ounces)
Berries, such as blueberries or raspberries (1 pint)
Garlic (1 head)
Lemons (2)
Limes (10)
Mixed salad greens (6 ounces)
Mushrooms (4 ounces)
Onion, red (1)
Onion, yellow, small (1)
Spinach (1 bunch)

DAIRY AND EGGS
Butter, unsalted (8 ounces)
Cheese, goat or feta, crumbled (4 ounces)
Cheese, Parmesan, shredded (8 ounces)
Cream cheese, full-fat (8 ounces)
Eggs, large (7)
Heavy cream (1 pint)
Yogurt, Greek, whole-milk, full-fat (17.6 ounces)

MEAT AND SEAFOOD
Beef, short ribs, boneless (1½ pounds; 3½ pounds if bone-in)
Chicken, thighs, boneless, skinless (1 pound)
Shrimp, medium, peeled and deveined (1 pound)

FROZEN
Spinach (1 [16-ounce] bag)

HERBS AND SPICES
Cinnamon, ground
Garlic powder
Peppercorns, black, ground
Salt, kosher
Thyme, dried

PANTRY
Almond milk, unsweetened (24 ounces)
Baking powder
Broth, beef (24 ounces)
Chia seeds
Coconut flakes, unsweetened
Coconut milk, full-fat, unsweetened (1 [13½-ounce] can)
Collagen peptides or other unsweetened protein powder
Flaxseed
Flour, almond
Macadamia nuts
Mayonnaise
Oil, olive, extra-virgin
Peanut butter, unsweetened
Sugar-free sweetener, such as Swerve
Tuna (4 [4-ounce] cans)
Vanilla extract
Vinegar, balsamic
Walnuts
Wine, red, dry (8 ounces)

PREP DAY #1

Estimated prep time: 55 minutes

1. Preheat the oven to 400°F.
2. Prepare two Overnight Smoothie Bowls (no berries). Store in airtight containers in the refrigerator.
3. Make the dressing for the Arugula Salad (step 1 of the recipe). Store covered in the refrigerator.
4. Prepare and bake the Baked Chicken Alfredo with Spinach. Once cool, transfer to individual serving containers to store in the fridge.
5. While the chicken bakes, make the Coconut-Nut Butter Power Balls. Store in the freezer.

PREP DAY #2

Estimated prep time: 30 minutes

1. Prepare the seafood and vegetables for the Simple Ceviche Salad (follow step 1 of the recipe). Store in airtight containers in the refrigerator.
2. Prepare the dressing for the Simple Ceviche Salad (step 2 of the recipe). Store in the refrigerator. When you are ready to serve the salad, follow step 3 to combine the prepared dressing with the seafood and vegetables.
3. Make the Creamy Avocado Dressing. Store covered in the refrigerator.

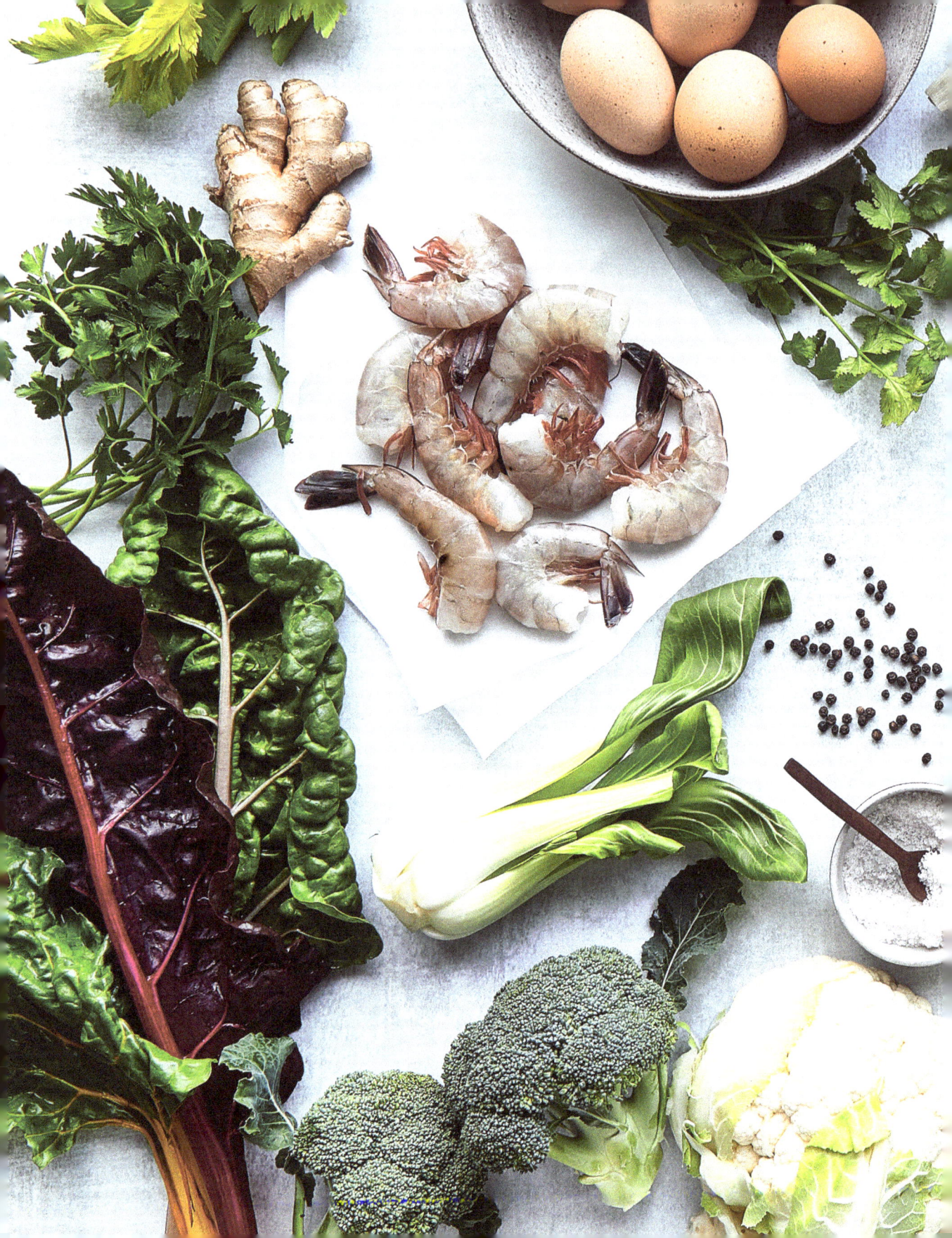

PART 2
KETO-FIT RECIPES

THE EASY AND FLAVOR-PACKED RECIPES in part 2 have been created with fitness enthusiasts in mind and will help you put the keto-fit lifestyle into practice. On their own, these recipes can complement any fitness routine, or you can use them as part of a more focused meal plan such as the ones laid out in chapter 3.

Both nutrition and fitness-focused labels are included on every recipe to highlight the power of the real-food ingredients included in each meal. Those marked "Overall Fitness" have balanced ketogenic ratios that can be used for any activity level and diet plan to provide a good mix of nutrients while maintaining ketosis. Those marked "Strength Training" include a slightly higher plant-based carbohydrate load to provide a burst of energy for more intense anaerobic activities while continuing to be keto fit–friendly. Recipes labeled "Cardio" have higher fat ratios to help with endurance through longer-lasting fuel from fats and ketones.

These healthy recipes contain a wide variety of spices and natural flavors and use minimal added sweeteners (always optional). I hope you learn to love coming up with your own flavor combinations as much as I do; I've noted substitution or variation suggestions to encourage your creative side. Have fun, fuel up, and enjoy your keto-fit journey!

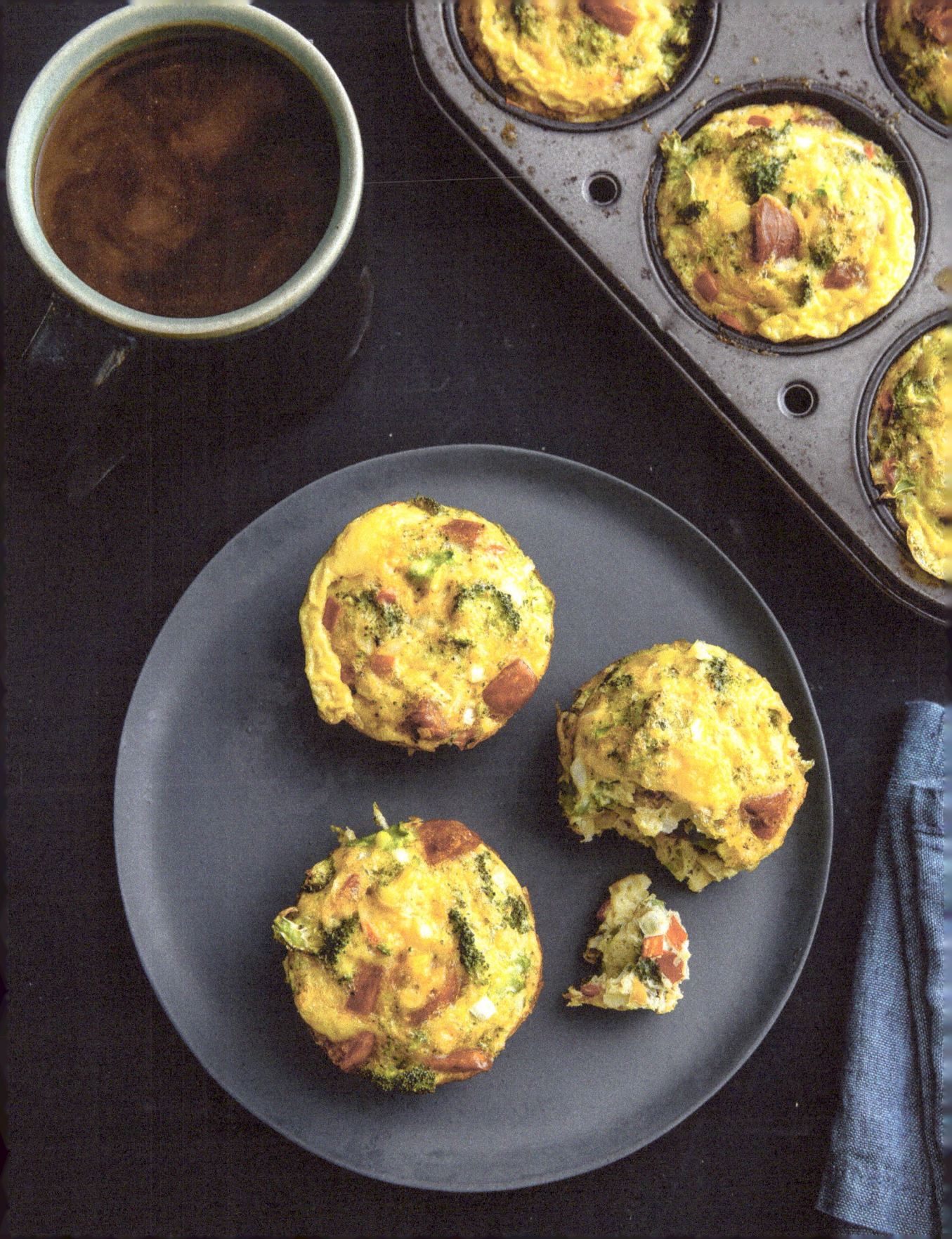

CHAPTER 4

Breakfast

Broccoli and Cheddar Mini Quiches 50

Fully-Fueled Protein Shake 51

Nutty Baked Oatmeal 52

Creamy Bacon-Egg Salad 53

Overnight Smoothie Bowl 54

Spinach Shakshuka 55

Breakfast Pizza 56

Broccoli and Cheddar Mini Quiches

OVERALL FITNESS

Serves 6

Prep time: 15 mins
Cook time: 20 mins

Eggs are a high-quality post-workout source of protein but don't always travel or reheat well. These little gems do both, making them an ideal part of weekly meal prep. Quiche is super versatile, so feel free to mix it up. I love replicating the flavors of spinach-artichoke dip using canned artichoke hearts, frozen spinach, and goat cheese for a tasty twist. The possibilities are endless!

Olive oil or butter, for coating the muffin tin
12 large eggs
1 teaspoon kosher salt
1 teaspoon garlic powder or 1 tablespoon minced fresh garlic
1 teaspoon onion powder
½ teaspoon freshly ground black pepper
½ teaspoon smoked paprika (optional)
2 cups thawed chopped frozen broccoli florets
1 cup shredded cheddar cheese
4 ounces cooked bacon, crumbled (optional)

1. Preheat the oven to 350°F. Coat the cups of a 12-count muffin tin with olive oil.
2. In a medium bowl, whisk together the eggs, salt, garlic powder, onion powder, pepper, and paprika (if using).
3. Whisk in the broccoli, cheese, and bacon (if using).
4. Divide the egg mixture evenly among the prepared muffin cups.
5. Transfer the muffin tin to the oven and bake for 18 to 20 minutes, or until the quiches are puffed up and cooked through. Remove from the oven. Let cool slightly. Serve warm.

▶ **STORAGE TIP:** Extra quiches can be cooled completely and stored in an airtight freezer bag in the freezer for up to 2 months or in the refrigerator for up to 1 week. Simply reheat in the microwave or oven before serving.

Per Serving (2 mini quiches): Calories: 460; Total fat: 32g; Total carbs: 8g; Fiber: 2g; Net carbs: 6g; Protein: 35g
Macros: 63% Fat; 30% Protein; 7% Carbs

Fully-Fueled Protein Shake

OVERALL FITNESS

Serves 1

Prep time: 5 mins

Quick and easy, protein shakes are a convenient way to get the amino acids your body needs after workouts to preserve and grow lean body mass and allow your muscles to recover. Unfortunately, so many store-bought options—although high in protein—lack the fat, to make them keto friendly and are often loaded with sugars. This high-fat, moderate-protein option uses collagen peptides as a protein source for the added bonus of gut-healing and tissue-repairing properties. Feel free to substitute your favorite sugar-free protein powder if you prefer, but stick to a 15-gram protein serving size.

- 1 cup full-fat canned coconut milk
- ½ cup unsweetened almond milk or ice, plus more as needed
- 2 tablespoons unsweetened peanut butter
- 1½ scoops unflavored collagen peptides
- 1 teaspoon vanilla extract
- 1 to 2 teaspoons granulated sugar-free sweetener, such as monk fruit or stevia (optional)

Put the coconut milk, almond milk, peanut butter, collagen peptides, vanilla, and sweetener (if using) in a blender or large wide-mouth jar (if using an immersion blender). Blend until smooth and creamy, adding more almond milk or ice to achieve your desired consistency. Serve cold.

▶ **STORAGE TIP:** Make this shake the night before and store in the refrigerator for grab-and-go early morning post-workout fuel. Shake well before serving.

Per Serving: Calories: 720; Total fat: 66g; Total carbs: 13g; Fiber: 4.5g; Net carbs: 8.5g; Protein: 18g
Macros: 83% Fat; 10% Protein; 7% Carbs

Nutty Baked Oatmeal

STRENGTH TRAINING

Serves 4

Prep time: 5 mins
Cook time: 40 mins

The small amount of oats in this recipe serves as a quick-acting source of glucose to power an intense strength workout. Steel-cut oats have a deep, nutty flavor and more fiber than traditional oats. Substitute traditional quick or rolled oats in an equal amount if you prefer.

- 1 tablespoon unsalted butter
- ½ cup unsweetened almond milk
- ¼ cup quick-cooking steel-cut oats
- 1 teaspoon ground cinnamon
- 1 teaspoon vanilla extract
- 4 large eggs
- ¼ cup ground flaxseed
- 1 teaspoon baking powder
- ½ cup coarsely chopped walnuts

1. Preheat the oven to 375°F. Coat the inside of an 8½-inch-by-4½-inch loaf pan with the butter.
2. In a small saucepan, bring the almond milk to a boil over high heat.
3. Add the oats. Reduce the heat to low. Simmer, stirring occasionally, for 5 to 6 minutes, or until thickened and the oats have cooked. Remove from the heat.
4. Stir in the cinnamon and vanilla.
5. In a large bowl, whisk together the eggs, flaxseed, and baking powder.
6. Add the oats, whisking constantly so that the heat does not cook the eggs.
7. Stir in the nuts and transfer the mixture to the prepared loaf pan.
8. Transfer the loaf pan to the oven and bake for 20 to 25 minutes, or until the oats have fully set in the middle and are golden brown on top. Remove from the oven. Let cool for 5 minutes before slicing.

▶ **STORAGE TIP:** This baked oatmeal will keep in an airtight container in the refrigerator for up to 1 week. Simply reheat in the microwave or oven prior to serving.

Per Serving: Calories: 269; Total fat: 20g; Total carbs: 11g; Fiber: 3.5g; Net carbs: 7.5g; Protein: 11.5g
Macros: 67% Fat; 17% Protein; 16% Carbs

Creamy Bacon-Egg Salad

CARDIO
Serves 4

Prep time: 15 mins, plus 1 hr to chill

Cook time: 20 mins

Egg salad is a simple way to incorporate a lot of extra fat into a portable meal. This version adds creamy avocado for fat, fiber, and potassium, plus the crunch of crispy bacon for a breakfast pairing made in heaven. Buy precooked hard-boiled eggs to make prep even quicker.

8 large eggs
¼ cup mayonnaise
1 ripe large avocado, pitted, peeled, and mashed
½ teaspoon kosher salt
¼ teaspoon freshly ground black pepper
1 tablespoon minced red onion (optional)
2 tablespoons chopped fresh parsley (optional)
4 bacon slices, cooked and crumbled

1. Bring a large pot of water to a boil over high heat.
2. Carefully place the eggs in the boiling water and boil for 15 minutes. Remove from the heat and immediately drain and run cool water over the eggs. Transfer to a bowl. Cover with ice or very cold water until cool to the touch. Then peel the eggs, coarsely chop, and put in a medium bowl.
3. In a large bowl, whisk together the mayonnaise, avocado, salt, and pepper.
4. Add the onion and parsley (if using). Stir until smooth.
5. Add the eggs and bacon. Stir until just combined. Refrigerate for 1 hour before serving.

▶ **STORAGE TIP:** Egg salad can be stored covered in the refrigerator for up to 2 days. The salad will become runny and the avocado will brown the longer it is stored; don't make more than you plan to eat within a couple days.

Per Serving: Calories: 331; Total fat: 28g; Total carbs: 4g; Fiber: 2.5g; Net carbs: 1.5g; Protein: 16g
Macros: 76% Fat; 19% Protein; 5% Carbs

Overnight Smoothie Bowl

CARDIO
STRENGTH TRAINING
Serves 1

Prep time: 5 mins, plus 8 to 12 hrs to chill

This convenient breakfast is a cross between a smoothie and chia pudding and will thicken the longer it sits in the refrigerator. It's a perfect keto-friendly combination of all three macronutrients: protein, fat, and healthy fast-acting carbs for heavy lifting or high-intensity workout days. To make this lower carb, omit the fruit entirely or cut the amount in half.

- ½ cup whole-milk plain Greek yogurt
- ¼ cup full-fat canned coconut milk or heavy cream
- 1 teaspoon vanilla extract
- 1 to 2 teaspoons granulated sugar-free sweetener, such as monk fruit or stevia (optional)
- ½ cup finely chopped strawberries (optional)
- 2 tablespoons chopped macadamia nuts
- 1 tablespoon chia seeds

1. In a Mason jar or small glass bowl with a lid, whisk together the yogurt, coconut milk, vanilla, and sweetener (if using) until smooth.

2. Add the strawberries (if using), nuts, and chia seeds. Stir to combine well. Cover tightly with a lid and refrigerate to thicken overnight.

▶ **STORAGE TIP:** Although this smoothie bowl will be ready to enjoy the next morning, it can be stored in the refrigerator for up to 4 days. Double or even quadruple the recipe to make several days' worth of easy on-the-go breakfasts or snacks.

Per Serving: Calories: 399; Total fat: 32g; Total carbs: 13g; Fiber: 5.5g; Net carbs: 7.5g; Protein: 15g
Macros: 72% Fat; 15% Protein; 13% Carbs

Spinach Shakshuka

OVERALL FITNESS

Serves 6

Prep time: 5 mins
Cook time: 25 mins

Shakshuka, eggs baked in spicy tomato sauce, is a brunch favorite. It may sound fancy but it is simple to make, and this keto-friendly version is full of quality micronutrients.

---

2 cups no-sugar-added marinara sauce, such as Rao's brand (look for less than 5g sugar per serving)

10 ounces frozen chopped spinach

½ cup plus 2 tablespoons extra-virgin olive oil

1 teaspoon garlic powder

1 to 2 teaspoons red pepper flakes (optional)

6 large eggs

6 ounces crumbled vegetarian feta or goat cheese

1. In a large deep skillet, combine the marinara sauce and spinach. Bring to a simmer over medium-high heat, stirring until the spinach is thawed and blends into the sauce.

2. Reduce the heat to medium-low. Stir in ½ cup of oil, the garlic powder, and red pepper flakes (if using). Cover the skillet with a lid or aluminum foil.

3. Reduce the heat to low. Simmer for 5 minutes, or until the mixture is very hot and fragrant.

4. Gently crack each egg into the simmering sauce, allowing each egg to create a crater. Do not allow the eggs to touch.

5. Sprinkle the eggs with the cheese. Cover the skillet and poach the eggs for 8 to 12 minutes, or until the yolks reach your desired consistency and the cheese has melted.

6. Drizzle with the remaining 2 tablespoons of oil. Remove from the heat. Serve warm.

▶ **STORAGE TIP:** Shakshuka is best when the eggs are freshly cooked. To prep ahead, make the sauce (steps 1 to 3). Cover and refrigerate for up to 4 days. When you are ready to eat, reheat the sauce in the skillet over medium-low heat, then follow steps 4 to 6.

Per Serving: Calories: 386; Total fat: 34.5g; Total carbs: 8g; Fiber: 2.5g; Net carbs: 5.5g; Protein: 12g

Macros: 80% Fat; 12% Protein; 8% Carbs

Breakfast Pizza

STRENGTH TRAINING

Serves 4

Prep time: 10 mins
Cook time: 25 mins

Who doesn't love pizza for breakfast? This high-protein keto-friendly version is the perfect recovery treat after a strenuous strength training workout. You can omit pepperoni and load the pizza with low-carb vegetables, such as mushrooms, peppers, or onions, if you prefer.

- ¼ cup extra-virgin olive oil
- 4 large eggs
- ¼ cup heavy cream
- 1½ cups shredded mozzarella cheese, divided
- 1 teaspoon kosher salt
- 1 teaspoon Italian seasoning or dried oregano or rosemary
- ¼ teaspoon freshly ground black pepper
- ½ teaspoon baking powder
- ½ cup no-sugar-added marinara sauce, such as Rao's (look for less than 5g sugar per serving)
- 4 ounces sliced pepperoni

1. Preheat the oven to 375°F. Drizzle the oil in an 8- or 9-inch pie pan or glass baking dish and swirl to coat. Alternatively, you can make a square pizza in an 8-by-8-inch glass baking dish.

2. In a medium bowl, whisk together the eggs, cream, ½ cup of cheese, the salt, Italian seasoning, pepper, and baking powder. Transfer to the prepared pie pan.

3. Transfer the pie pan to the oven and bake for 10 to 15 minutes, or until the eggs are just set. Remove from the oven, leaving the oven on.

4. Spread the marinara sauce on top of the baked eggs.

5. Top with the remaining 1 cup of cheese and the pepperoni. Return the pie pan to the oven and bake for 8 to 10 minutes, or until the cheese has melted and the pepperoni is crispy. Remove from the oven. Let rest for 5 minutes before slicing.

▶ **STORAGE TIP:** Cooked pizza will store in the refrigerator for up to 4 days. Simply slice and reheat in the microwave or in the oven at 350°F before serving.

Per Serving: Calories: 513; Total fat: 45g; Total carbs: 5g; Fiber: 0.5g; Net carbs: 4.5g; Protein: 22g
Macros: 79% Fat; 17% Protein; 4% Carbs

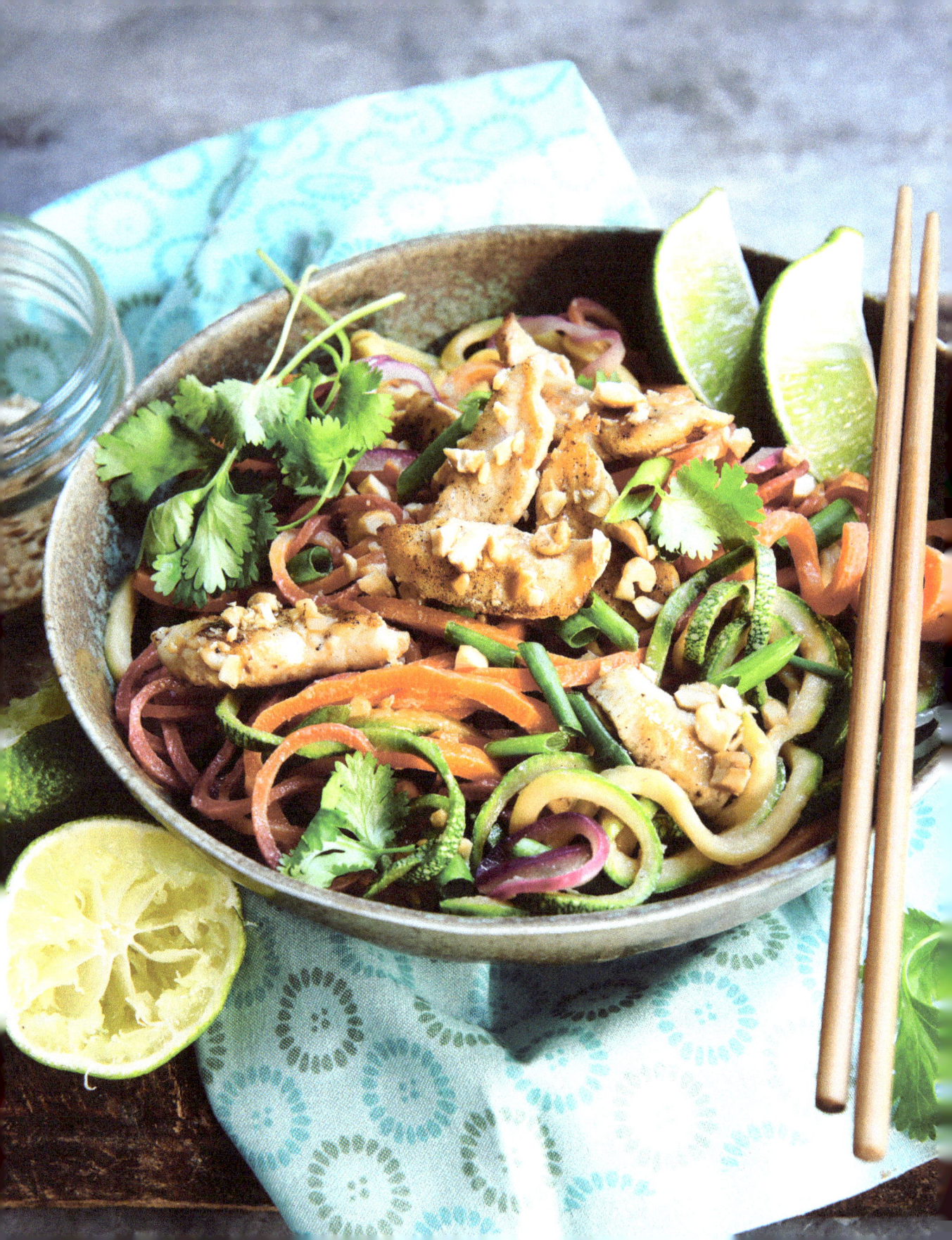

CHAPTER 5

Vegetables and Sides

Fuel Up Arugula Salad 60

Zucchini Tots 61

Asparagus Benedict 62

Shaved Brussels Hash 63

Guacamole Salad 64

Easy Greek Salad 65

Riced Cauliflower and Herb Salad 66

Peanut and Lime Zoodles 67

Fuel Up Arugula Salad

OVERALL FITNESS

Serves 4

Prep time: 10 mins

Arugula, a tender green with a slightly peppery flavor, is one of the top 20 nutrient-dense foods with a very high vitamin and mineral content in relation to its caloric value. It is my go-to salad green for maximum bang for your buck, but feel free to substitute baby kale or spinach in this salad if you prefer. This simple salad is packed with other great macronutrients: healthy fats from seeds, nuts, and olive oil and protein from the cheese. Boost the protein by serving this salad alongside leftover fish, chicken, or steak.

¼ cup extra-virgin olive oil
Grated zest and juice of 1 lemon (2 to 3 tablespoons)
1 tablespoon balsamic vinegar
½ teaspoon kosher salt
8 cups baby arugula
1 cup coarsely chopped walnuts
4 ounces crumbled vegetarian feta or goat cheese
¼ cup roasted pumpkin seeds (optional)

1. To make the dressing, in a small bowl, whisk together the oil, lemon zest, lemon juice, vinegar, and salt.
2. In a large bowl, combine the arugula, walnuts, cheese, and pumpkin seeds (if using).
3. Drizzle with the dressing and toss to coat. Serve immediately.

▶ **STORAGE TIP:** Once dressed, this salad does not keep long in the refrigerator. You can prep all the ingredients ahead, including the dressing, and store the salad and dressing in separate containers in the refrigerator for up to 4 days. Toss together just before serving.

Per Serving: Calories: 412; Total fat: 37g; Total carbs: 9.5g; Fiber: 3g; Net carbs: 6.5g; Protein: 10g
Macros: 81% Fat; 10% Protein; 9% Carbs

Zucchini Tots

OVERALL FITNESS
Serves 4

Prep time: 25 mins
Cook time: 20 mins

These crispy tots are a fun side served with the Easy Slow-Cooked Ribs (page 84). Use a box grater or food processor to grate the zucchini and don't skip the draining step. Zucchini is naturally loaded with water; if it isn't drained, you'll get soggy tots that fall apart.

- 4 tablespoons extra-virgin olive oil, divided
- 2 cups shredded zucchini (about 2 medium zucchini)
- 1½ teaspoons kosher salt, divided
- 1 large egg, beaten
- ½ cup shredded cheddar cheese
- ½ cup almond flour
- 1 teaspoon baking powder
- ¼ teaspoon freshly ground black pepper

1. Preheat the oven to 400°F. Line a baking sheet with aluminum foil, drizzle with 2 tablespoons of oil, and spread evenly. Line a colander with paper towels.
2. Put the zucchini in the prepared colander and sprinkle with ½ teaspoon of salt. Top with another layer of paper towels and let sit for 10 minutes. Press down on the zucchini to release excess water and pat dry.
3. In a large bowl, combine the zucchini, remaining 1 teaspoon of salt, the egg, cheese, almond flour, baking powder, and pepper.
4. Spoon 2 tablespoons of the mixture into your hands and roll into small ovals. The mixture will be sticky. Put the ovals on the prepared baking sheet. Drizzle with the remaining 2 tablespoons of oil.
5. Transfer the baking sheet to the oven and bake, turning halfway through cooking, for 15 to 20 minutes, or until the tots are set and golden brown. Remove from the oven.

▶ **STORAGE TIP:** Cooked tots will keep in the refrigerator covered for up to 4 days. Reheat in the oven at 400°F on a foil-lined baking sheet until crispy and heated through.

Per Serving: Calories: 276; Total fat: 25g; Total carbs: 4g; Fiber: 2g; Net carbs: 2g; Protein: 8g
Macros: 82% Fat; 12% Protein; 6% Carbs

Asparagus Benedict

CARDIO

Serves 6

Prep time: 5 mins
Cook time: 25 mins

- 1 pound fresh asparagus, trimmed
- 6 tablespoons olive oil, divided
- 1 teaspoon kosher salt
- ¼ teaspoon freshly ground black pepper
- 1 cup heavy cream
- 1 (0.9-ounce) packet Hollandaise sauce mix, such as Knorr
- 6 tablespoons unsalted butter
- 6 large eggs

1. Preheat the oven to 425°F. Line a baking sheet with aluminum foil.
2. In a large bowl, drizzle the asparagus with 2 tablespoons of oil, the salt, and pepper. Toss to coat. Arrange the asparagus in a single layer on the prepared baking sheet.
3. Transfer the baking sheet to the oven and roast for 18 to 20 minutes, or until the asparagus is tender but not mushy. Remove from the oven. Divide among 6 plates.
4. Meanwhile, in a small saucepan, whisk together the cream and Hollandaise mix. Bring to a boil over high heat, whisking constantly. Add the butter and whisk until smooth.
5. Reduce the heat to low. Simmer, whisking constantly, for 1 to 2 minutes, or until the sauce is thick and creamy. Remove from the heat. Cover and keep warm.
6. In a large skillet, heat 2 tablespoons of oil over medium-high heat. Crack 3 eggs into the skillet and fry for 2 minutes, or until just set.
7. Flip the eggs and cook for 1 to 2 minutes for a runny yolk or 3 to 4 minutes for a set yolk. Remove the eggs from the skillet. Keep warm. Repeat with the remaining 2 tablespoons of oil and 3 eggs.
8. Drizzle each serving with 3 tablespoons of sauce and top with a fried egg.

▶ **STORAGE TIP:** The sauce can be made ahead and stored covered in the refrigerator for up to 4 days. Reheat and whisk well before serving.

Per Serving: Calories: 453; Total fat: 44g; Total carbs: 6.5g; Fiber: 1g; Net carbs: 5.5g; Protein: 8g
Macros: 87% Fat; 7% Protein; 6% Carbs

Shaved Brussels Hash

OVERALL FITNESS

Serves 4

Prep time: 15 mins
Cook time: 20 mins

Crispy delicate Brussels sprouts loaded with bacon? Yes, please! If you have a food processor, using the slicing blade makes shaving the Brussels a breeze, but slicing them by hand is also a great option. You can replicate all the flavor with simply halved or quartered sprouts, but it will have less of a hash consistency.

---

4 tablespoons extra-virgin olive oil, divided
8 ounces bacon, chopped
1 pound Brussels sprouts, very thinly sliced lengthwise
¼ cup chopped red onion
4 garlic cloves, minced
1 teaspoon dried thyme
½ teaspoon kosher salt
¼ teaspoon freshly ground black pepper
¼ cup chopped Italian parsley leaves (optional)

1. In a large deep skillet, heat 2 tablespoons of oil over medium heat.
2. Add the bacon and fry for 5 to 6 minutes, or until crispy. Using a slotted spoon, remove the cooked bacon, leaving the rendered fat in the skillet and set aside.
3. Add the remaining 2 tablespoons of oil to the skillet and heat over medium heat.
4. Add the Brussels sprouts and onion. Fry, stirring constantly, for 5 to 6 minutes, or until tender and lightly browned.
5. Add the garlic, thyme, salt, and pepper. Sauté for 2 to 3 minutes. Remove from the heat.
6. Stir in the bacon and parsley (if using). Serve warm.

▶ **STORAGE TIP:** The cooked hash will store covered in the refrigerator for up to 4 days. To crisp back up, place in a hot skillet and fry until crispy and heated through.

Per Serving: Calories: 404; Total fat: 35g; Total carbs: 11g; Fiber: 4g; Net carbs: 7g; Protein: 11g
Macros: 78% Fat; 11% Protein; 11% Carbs

Guacamole Salad

CARDIO
Serves 4

Prep time: 10 mins

This easy salad is like a deconstructed bowl of guacamole, without the need for chips! High in heart-healthy fats with the addition of olive oil and roasted pumpkin seeds, it is great for sustained ketogenic energy for those longer cardio workouts. Add some grilled chicken, shrimp, or meat for a quick complete weeknight dinner.

- 2 ripe large avocados, pitted, peeled, and cut into 1-inch chunks
- ½ cup cherry tomatoes, halved
- ½ cup packed fresh cilantro leaves
- ¼ cup chopped scallions, green and white parts
- 1 or 2 jalapeño peppers, seeded and chopped (optional)
- ¼ cup extra-virgin olive oil
- Juice of 1 lemon
- 1 teaspoon kosher salt
- ¼ teaspoon freshly ground black pepper
- 2 tablespoons roasted pumpkin seeds (optional)

1. To make the salad, in a medium bowl, combine the avocados, tomatoes, cilantro, scallions, and jalapeño (if using).

2. In a small bowl, whisk together the oil, lemon juice, salt, and pepper. Drizzle over the salad.

3. Add the pumpkin seeds (if using) and toss to coat. Serve immediately or chill.

▶ **STORAGE TIP:** Avocados naturally brown when they are oxidized, but the lemon juice will slow this process. You can also delay browning by making sure the salad is covered with plastic wrap that touches the surface of the food and is sealed tightly so that no air reaches the salad. Covered properly, this salad will store in the refrigerator for up to 4 days.

Per Serving: Calories: 256; Total fat: 24g; Total carbs: 8g; Fiber: 5g; Net carbs: 3g; Protein: 2g
Macros: 84% Fat; 3% Protein; 13% Carbs

Easy Greek Salad

OVERALL FITNESS

Serves 4

Prep time: 10 mins

Just when you think you've gotten sick of salads, this simple Greek salad kicks up the flavor. Full of omega-3 rich healthy fats, this salad is a Mediterranean diet staple. Add grilled chicken, nuts, or sliced hard-boiled egg for a higher-protein post-workout meal.

- 8 cups coarsely chopped romaine lettuce
- 4 roma tomatoes, chopped
- 1 large cucumber, ends removed, cut lengthwise and then into half-moons
- 20 Kalamata olives, pitted and halved
- ¼ red onion, thinly sliced
- 4 ounces crumbled vegetarian feta cheese
- ½ cup extra-virgin olive oil
- Juice of 1 lemon (2 to 3 tablespoons)
- 1 teaspoon dried oregano or Greek seasoning
- ½ teaspoon kosher salt
- ¼ teaspoon freshly ground black pepper

1. To make the salad, in a large bowl, combine the lettuce, tomatoes, cucumber, olives, onion, and cheese.
2. To make the dressing, in a small bowl, whisk together the oil, lemon juice, oregano, salt, and pepper.
3. Add the dressing to the salad and toss to coat.

▶ **STORAGE TIP:** I love to prep these for the week in Mason jars to make storage and transport a breeze. If prepping ahead, place tomatoes and cucumbers at the bottom to protect the lighter vegetables and lettuce from getting soggy in storage and toss with the dressing just before serving.

Per Serving: Calories: 410; Total fat: 38g; Total carbs: 11g; Fiber: 3.5g; Net carbs: 7.5g; Protein: 6g
Macros: 83% Fat; 6% Protein; 11% Carbs

Riced Cauliflower and Herb Salad

OVERALL FITNESS

Serves 6

Prep time: 15 mins, plus 30 mins to chill

Cook time: 5 mins

This dish is a low-carb spin on tabbouleh, a grain-based side dish common in Middle Eastern cuisine. I find that fresh riced cauliflower—made at home on a box grater or in the food processor—has superior texture, but feel free to use prepared options as well.

- 6 tablespoons extra-virgin olive oil, divided
- 4 cups riced cauliflower (thawed and drained if using frozen)
- 2 garlic cloves, minced
- 1½ teaspoons kosher salt
- ¼ teaspoon freshly ground black pepper
- ½ cup chopped fresh mint
- ½ cup chopped fresh Italian parsley
- ½ cup chopped celery
- ¼ cup minced red onion
- ½ cup diced red bell pepper
- Juice of 1 lemon (2 to 3 tablespoons)
- 2 ripe large avocados, peeled, pitted, and diced

1. In a large skillet, heat 2 tablespoons of oil over medium-high heat.
2. Add the riced cauliflower, garlic, salt, and black pepper. Sauté for 3 to 4 minutes, or until tender but not mushy. Remove from the heat. Transfer to a large bowl.
3. Toss in the mint, parsley, celery, onion, and bell pepper.
4. In a small bowl, whisk together the remaining 4 tablespoons of oil and the lemon juice. Drizzle over the vegetables and toss to coat.
5. Gently stir in the avocado, being careful not to mash it. Refrigerate the salad uncovered (to allow any steam to escape) for at least 30 minutes before serving.

▶ **STORAGE TIP:** Dressed, this salad will store in the refrigerator for 1 day before getting soggy. To prep further out, complete steps 1 to 3 and refrigerate covered for up to 4 days. Toss with dressing and avocado just prior to serving.

Per Serving: Calories: 232; Total fat: 20g; Total carbs: 10g; Fiber: 5.5g; Net carbs: 4.5g; Protein: 3g
Macros: 78% Fat; 5% Protein; 17% Carbs

Peanut and Lime Zoodles

OVERALL FITNESS
Serves 4

Prep time: 15 mins
Cook time: 15 mins

The secret to "al dente" zoodles (zucchini noodles) is to keep them raw and toss with a warm sauce. Fresh zucchini is the only way to make this work; frozen options wilt quickly.

- ½ cup unsweetened peanut butter
- ¼ cup tamari or soy sauce (if not gluten-free)
- 2 tablespoons toasted sesame oil
- 2 tablespoons freshly squeezed lime juice (from about 2 limes)
- 1 tablespoon sriracha or other hot sauce (optional)
- 1 to 2 teaspoons granulated sugar-free sweetener, such as monk fruit or stevia (optional)
- 1 teaspoon ground ginger
- 2 tablespoons olive oil
- 1 red bell pepper, cored and thinly sliced
- 1 cup broccoli florets, cut into bite-size pieces
- 8 ounces mushrooms, sliced
- 4 garlic cloves, minced
- 4 cups spiralized fresh zucchini (from about 2 medium zucchini)

1. To make the sauce, in a small bowl, whisk together the peanut butter, tamari, sesame oil, lime juice, sriracha (if using), sweetener (if using), and ginger.
2. In a large skillet, heat the olive oil over medium-high heat.
3. Add the bell pepper and broccoli. Sauté for 2 minutes, or until the vegetables are slightly softened.
4. Add the mushrooms and sauté for 6 to 8 minutes, or until the vegetables are tender but not mushy.
5. Add the garlic and sauce. Sauté, stirring well to combine, for 1 to 2 minutes, or until smooth. Remove from the heat.
6. In a large bowl, combine the hot vegetables, sauce, and zucchini. Toss to coat. Serve warm.

▶ **STORAGE TIP:** This dish will keep covered in the refrigerator for up to 4 days. Serve leftovers cold; they are delicious that way, and reheating will cause the zucchini to lose its "al dente" bite.

Per Serving: Calories: 400; Total fat: 32g; Total carbs: 16g; Fiber: 4g; Net carbs: 12g; Protein: 12g
Macros: 72% Fat; 12% Protein; 16% Carbs

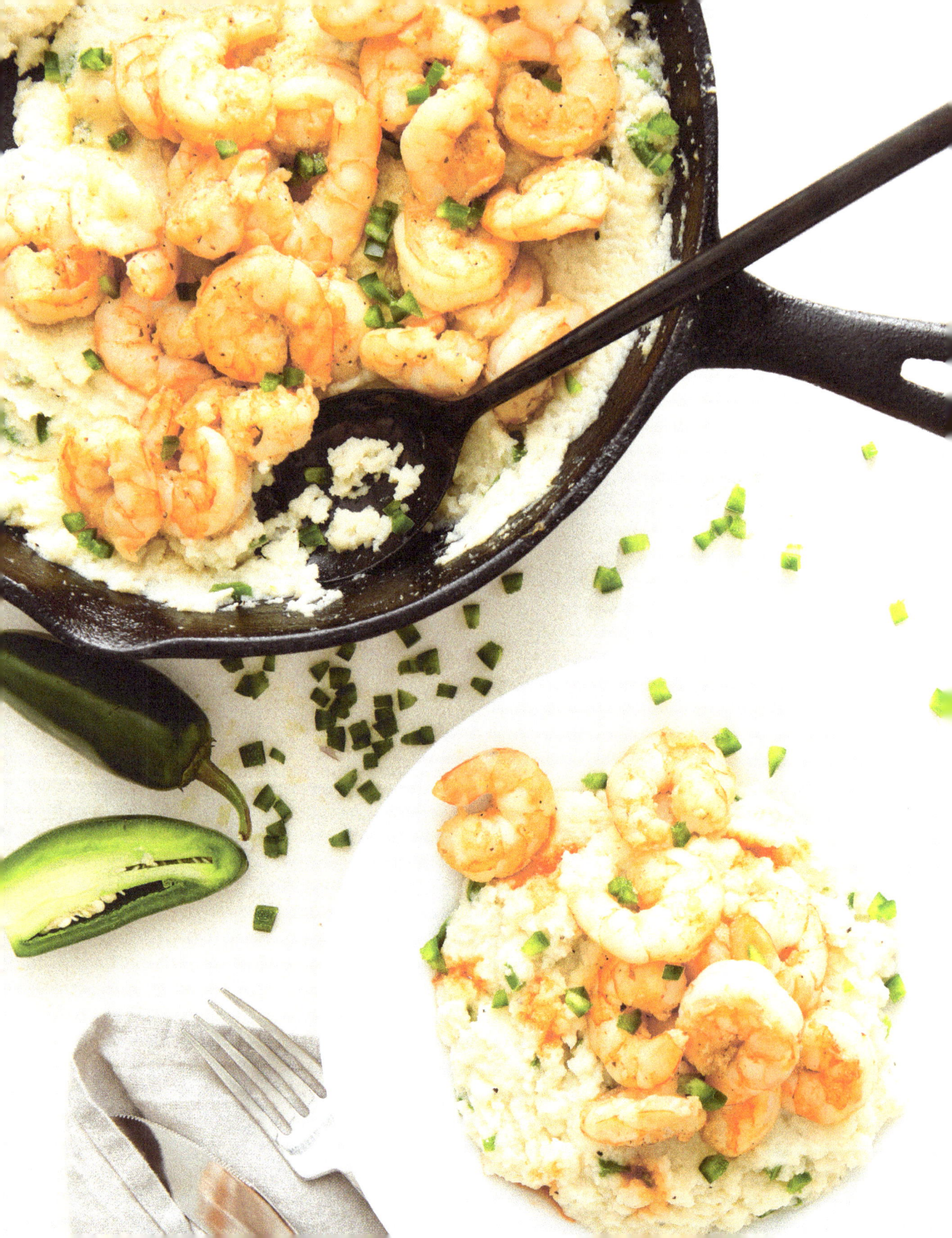

CHAPTER 6

Seafood and Poultry

Shrimp and Creamy Cauliflower "Grits" 70

Herby Orange Baked Chicken 71

Parmesan Chicken Meatball Casserole 72

Spiced Chicken Wings and Brussels 73

Nigiri-Inspired Salmon and Avocado 74

Slow Cooker Chicken Tikka Masala 75

Fish Tacos in Lettuce Boats 76

Simple Ceviche Salad 77

Baked Chicken Alfredo with Spinach 78

Greek Stuffed Chicken Breasts 79

Shrimp and Creamy Cauliflower "Grits"

OVERALL FITNESS

Serves 4

Prep time: 15 mins
Cook time: 20 mins

In this variation on a Southern favorite, riced cauliflower mimics traditional cheesy grits. It's wonderful as a dinner or a heavy brunch, as is common in Southern cuisine.

FOR THE CREAMY CAULIFLOWER

8 ounces full-fat cream cheese
¼ cup heavy cream
4 tablespoons (½ stick) unsalted butter, divided
1 teaspoon kosher salt
¼ teaspoon freshly ground black pepper
2 cups fresh or frozen riced cauliflower
½ cup shredded cheddar cheese

FOR THE SHRIMP

¼ cup extra-virgin olive oil
1 pound shrimp, peeled and deveined
4 garlic cloves, minced
1 teaspoon kosher salt
¼ teaspoon freshly ground black pepper
1 jalapeño, diced (optional)
Shredded cheddar cheese, for garnish (optional)

1. **To make the creamy cauliflower:** In a medium saucepan, combine the cream cheese, cream, 2 tablespoons of butter, the salt, and pepper. Bring to just below a boil over high heat, whisking to blend.
2. When the mixture is smooth, add the riced cauliflower.
3. Reduce the heat to low. Simmer, stirring occasionally, for 8 to 10 minutes, or until the cauliflower is tender and most of the water has evaporated. Remove from the heat.
4. Stir in the cheese and remaining 2 tablespoons of butter. Keep warm.
5. **To make the shrimp:** In a medium skillet, heat the oil over medium heat.
6. Add the shrimp, garlic, salt, and pepper. Sauté for 2 to 3 minutes, or until the shrimp are pink and cooked through. Remove from the heat.
7. Serve the shrimp over the cauliflower "grits," garnished with the jalapeño (if using) and more cheese (if using).

▶ **STORAGE TIP:** Both the shrimp and cauliflower mixtures will store well covered (in separate containers) in the refrigerator for up to 4 days.

Per Serving: Calories: 620; Total fat: 54.5g; Total carbs: 7g; Fiber: 1g; Net carbs: 6g; Protein: 25g
Macros: 79% Fat; 16% Protein; 5% Carbs

Herby Orange Baked Chicken

STRENGTH TRAINING

Serves 4

Prep time: 5 mins
Cook time: 30 mins

These chicken thighs are my go-to for a quick weeknight meal so rich in flavor my family raves every time. They are delicious served as leftovers atop mixed greens. Or you can even shred them and combine them with some quality mayonnaise and a handful of sliced almonds for a chicken salad that is a great source of protein after a strength workout.

1¼ pounds boneless skinless chicken thighs
2 tablespoons fresh thyme, rosemary, or oregano, or 2 teaspoons dried

1 teaspoon kosher salt
¼ teaspoon freshly ground black pepper
6 garlic cloves, peeled and smashed
½ red onion, thinly sliced

1 medium orange, unpeeled and sliced
¼ cup extra-virgin olive oil

1. Preheat the oven to 425°F.
2. Put the chicken in an 8-by-8-inch glass baking dish. Sprinkle with the thyme, salt, and pepper.
3. Spread the garlic and onion evenly atop the chicken.
4. Spread the orange slices over the vegetables. Drizzle with the oil.
5. Transfer the baking dish to the oven and roast, flipping halfway through, for 25 to 30 minutes, or until the chicken has cooked through. Remove from the oven. Discard the orange slices.
6. Serve the chicken warm, drizzled with the cooking juices and garnished with the onion and garlic if desired.

▶ **STORAGE TIP:** This chicken makes for great leftovers and will store in the refrigerator covered for up to 1 week. Reheat in the microwave or oven, or serve cold.

Per Serving: Calories: 308; Total fat: 19g; Total carbs: 5g; Fiber: 0.5g; Net carbs: 4.5g; Protein: 29g
Macros: 56% Fat; 38% Protein; 6% Carbs

Parmesan Chicken Meatball Casserole

OVERALL FITNESS
Serves 4

Prep time: 15 mins
Cook time: 25 mins

Chicken parm meets spaghetti and meatballs in this deliciously easy casserole. Serve as an appetizer to feed a larger group, or for a main meal, serve over spiralized zucchini (zoodles) or alongside a large tossed salad.

---

1 pound ground dark meat chicken (not lean)
1 cup shredded Parmesan cheese, divided
½ cup extra-virgin olive oil, divided
¼ cup almond flour

2 teaspoons dried oregano
1 teaspoon garlic powder
1 teaspoon kosher salt
¼ teaspoon freshly ground black pepper

2 cups no-sugar-added marinara sauce, such as Rao's brand (look for less than 5g sugar per serving), divided
1 cup shredded fresh mozzarella cheese

1. Preheat the oven to 375°F.
2. In a large bowl, combine the chicken, ½ cup of Parmesan cheese, ¼ cup of oil, the almond flour, oregano, garlic powder, salt, and pepper. Mix until well incorporated.
3. Spread 1 cup of marinara sauce over the bottom of an 8-by-8-inch glass baking dish.
4. Using your hands, form the mixture into 12 balls, 1½ to 2 inches in diameter. Place atop the layer of sauce.
5. Top with the remaining 1 cup of sauce, the mozzarella cheese, and remaining ½ cup of Parmesan cheese. Drizzle with the remaining ¼ cup of oil. Cover with aluminum foil.
6. Transfer the baking dish to the oven and bake for 18 to 20 minutes, or until the meatballs have cooked through and the sauce and cheese are bubbly.
7. Remove the foil. Bake for 5 more minutes, or until the cheese has lightly browned. Remove from the oven. Let rest for 5 minutes before serving.

▶ **STORAGE TIP:** Store this covered in the refrigerator for 4 days. You can also prep the meatballs ahead and assemble the casserole just prior to baking.

Per Serving: Calories: 609; Total fat: 46g; Total carbs: 12g; Fiber: 3g; Net carbs: 9g; Protein: 36g
Macros: 68% Fat; 24% Protein; 8% Carbs

Spiced Chicken Wings and Brussels

OVERALL FITNESS

Serves 4

Prep time: 15 mins
Cook time: 45 mins

With mostly hands-off cooking time, sheet pan dinners like this one are a breeze.

¼ cup extra-virgin olive oil
Grated zest and juice of 1 lemon
1 teaspoon kosher salt
1 teaspoon garlic powder
1 teaspoon ground cumin
1 teaspoon paprika
1 teaspoon ground allspice
½ to 1 teaspoon red pepper flakes (optional)
2 pounds bone-in chicken wings, split
1 pound Brussels sprouts, trimmed and quartered
Chopped cilantro or mint leaves, for serving (optional)

1. Preheat the oven to 450°F. Line a rimmed baking sheet with aluminum foil.
2. In a small bowl, whisk together the oil, lemon zest, lemon juice, salt, garlic powder, cumin, paprika, allspice, and red pepper flakes (if using).
3. Put the chicken in a large bowl and drizzle with half of the oil mixture. Toss to coat. Place the wings in a single layer on the prepared baking sheet. Set the bowl aside.
4. Transfer the baking sheet to the oven and roast for 20 minutes, or until the skin starts to brown and crisp.
5. Reduce the oven temperature to 425°F. Put the Brussels sprouts in the reserved bowl. (We will be cooking these so no need to wash the bowl.) Drizzle with the remaining oil mixture and toss to coat.
6. Remove the baking sheet from the oven. Arrange the Brussels sprouts in a single layer around the chicken.
7. Return the baking sheet to the oven and roast for 20 to 25 minutes, or until the chicken has cooked through and the Brussels sprouts are browned and crispy. Remove from the oven.
8. Sprinkle with cilantro (if using). Serve warm.

▶ **STORAGE TIP:** Store in an airtight container in the refrigerator for up to 4 days. Reheat on a foil-lined baking sheet in a 375°F oven until crisp.

Per Serving: Calories: 435; Total fat: 31g; Total carbs: 10g; Fiber: 4g; Net carbs: 6g; Protein: 29g
Macros: 64% Fat; 27% Protein; 9% Carbs

Nigiri-Inspired Salmon and Avocado

OVERALL FITNESS

Serves 4

Prep time: 10 mins

With all the flavor of sushi but none of the heavy carbs, these quick and easy snacks will satisfy your craving with minimal prep. This recipe is served open face like nigiri, rather than rolled like maki, and is fun to feed a crowd as an appetizer or serve as a lighter lunch. Roasted seaweed snacks can be found at most grocery stores in the international foods or snack aisle.

- 2 ripe large avocados, pitted and peeled
- 2 tablespoons toasted sesame oil
- 2 tablespoons olive oil
- 1 tablespoon tamari
- 16 (1½-by-2-inch) sheets roasted seaweed snacks (about 2 packs, depending on the brand)
- 8 ounces smoked salmon, chopped
- ⅛ teaspoon sriracha or other hot sauce (optional)

1. In a medium bowl, combine the avocados, sesame oil, olive oil, and tamari. Using a fork, mash well until smooth and creamy.
2. Lay the individual pieces of roasted seaweed snacks on a large cutting board or clean surface.
3. Top each with 2 tablespoons of the avocado mixture, followed by ½ ounce (about 1 tablespoon) of chopped salmon.
4. Top with the sriracha (if using). Serve immediately.

▶ **STORAGE TIP:** Once constructed, these snacks need to be served immediately. The avocado mixture and salmon can be prepped in advance and stored separately in the refrigerator, covered completely, for up to 2 days for a quick-assembly snack.

Per Serving: Calories: 323; Total fat: 27g; Total carbs: 7g; Fiber: 5g; Net carbs: 2g; Protein: 13g
Macros: 75% Fat; 16% Protein; 9% Carbs

Slow Cooker Chicken Tikka Masala

CARDIO
Serves 8

Prep time: 10 mins
Cook time: 10 mins, plus 4 to 5 hrs inactive time

Slow-cooked meals are my go-to for batch-cooking proteins throughout the week. If you don't have a slow cooker, simmer this covered on the stovetop in a large pot or Dutch oven over very low heat for 45 minutes to 1 hour. This recipe makes enough for eight servings; consider freezing leftover portions in individual containers.

---

8 tablespoons (1 stick) unsalted butter
½ yellow onion, finely chopped
1 (2-inch) piece fresh ginger, finely chopped, or 2 teaspoons ground ginger

8 garlic cloves, minced, or ¼ cup minced garlic
1 teaspoon kosher salt
2 tablespoons curry powder
2 (13½-ounce) cans full-fat coconut milk

¼ cup no-sugar-added tomato paste
2 pounds boneless skinless chicken thighs, cut into 1-inch chunks
Riced cauliflower or steamed frozen spinach, for serving

1. In a large skillet or saucepan, melt the butter over medium heat.
2. Add the onion and ginger. Sauté for 5 minutes, or until softened.
3. Add the garlic, salt, and curry powder. Sauté for 2 minutes, or until very fragrant.
4. Add the coconut milk and tomato paste. Whisk until smooth.
5. Increase the heat to high. Bring the mixture to just below a boil. Remove from the heat.
6. Put the chicken in the slow cooker and pour the sauce mixture over the chicken. Stir to coat. Cover with the lid and cook on low for 4 to 5 hours, or until the chicken is very tender. Turn off the slow cooker.
7. Serve the chicken and sauce mixture warm over riced cauliflower or steamed frozen spinach.

▶ **STORAGE TIP:** Store leftovers covered in the refrigerator for up to 4 days. This dish also freezes well and will keep in the freezer for up to 3 months.

Per Serving: Calories: 446; Total fat: 36g; Total carbs: 6g; Fiber: 2.5g; Net carbs: 4.5g; Protein: 25g
Macros: 73% Fat; 22% Protein; 5% Carbs

Fish Tacos in Lettuce Boats

OVERALL FITNESS
Serves 4

Prep time: 15 mins
Cook time: 10 mins

Taco Tuesday doesn't have to be a thing of the past just because you're going keto fit! The xanthan gum is optional in the flour "breading" but helps create a crispier coating.

- ½ cup sour cream
- 1 tablespoon freshly squeezed lime juice
- 1½ teaspoons kosher salt, divided
- ⅓ cup coconut flour
- 1 teaspoon xanthan gum (optional)
- 1 to 2 teaspoons chili powder
- 1 pound cod fillets or other white flaky fish, cut into 3-by-½-inch strips
- ¼ cup extra-virgin olive oil
- 8 Bibb lettuce or romaine lettuce leaves
- 2 ripe large avocados, pitted, peeled, and thinly sliced
- ¼ red onion, very thinly sliced
- 1 small jalapeño, seeded and thinly sliced (optional)
- ½ cup chopped fresh cilantro (optional)

1. In a small bowl, whisk together the sour cream, lime juice, and 1 teaspoon of salt.
2. In a large zip-top bag, combine the coconut flour, xanthan gum (if using), remaining ½ teaspoon of salt, and the chili powder. Shake well.
3. Add the fillets to the bag and shake to coat.
4. In a large skillet, heat the oil over medium-high heat.
5. When the oil is very hot, shake off excess flour from the fillets and transfer to the oil. Fry, turning frequently, for 4 to 6 minutes, or until golden and crispy. Turn off the heat. Using a slotted spoon or tongs, remove the fillets from the skillet and keep warm.
6. To serve, top each lettuce leaf with the fillets, avocado, onion, and 1 tablespoon of the sour cream mixture.
7. Garnish with the jalapeño (if using) and cilantro (if using).

▶ **STORAGE TIP:** Store in the refrigerator for up to 4 days. Reheat in a 400°F oven and assemble the lettuce boats just before serving.

Per Serving: Calories: 423; Total fat: 31g; Total carbs: 14g; Fiber: 9g; Net carbs: 5g; Protein: 22g
Macros: 66% Fat; 21% Protein; 13% Carbs

Simple Ceviche Salad

STRENGTH TRAINING

Serves 4

Prep time: 20 mins, plus 2 hrs to marinate

Ceviche, native to Peru, is a dish of seafood "cooked" in citrus juices without heating. Here, I cut the shrimp in half to reduce marinating time to 2 hours. If you prefer shrimp whole, increase the time they marinate to 6 to 8 hours (don't exceed 8 hours, or the shrimp will become tough). Serve this high-protein salad atop a bed of mixed greens.

- 1 pound medium shrimp, peeled, deveined, and cut in half lengthwise
- ½ small red onion, cut into thin slivers
- ¼ cup chopped fresh cilantro (optional)
- 1 medium jalapeño, seeded and sliced (optional)
- ⅓ cup freshly squeezed lime juice
- 2 tablespoons freshly squeezed lemon juice
- ½ cup extra-virgin olive oil
- 1 teaspoon kosher salt
- 2 ripe large avocados, peeled, pitted, and cut into ½-inch chunks

1. In a large glass bowl or Mason jar with a lid (metal bowls give the shrimp an "off" flavor), combine the shrimp, onion, cilantro (if using), and jalapeño (if using).

2. To make the dressing, in a small bowl, whisk together the lime juice, lemon juice, oil, and salt.

3. Add the dressing to the shrimp and toss well to coat. Cover and refrigerate for at least 2 hours. Give the mixture a toss every 30 minutes to make sure the shrimp continue to be coated in the juices.

4. Add the avocado just before serving and toss to combine.

▶ **STORAGE TIP:** To store leftovers or make this in advance, omit the olive oil when preparing the marinade. After marinating, drain all the citrus from the shrimp mixture. Then, add the olive oil, toss to coat, and store in the refrigerator for up to 4 days. Add the avocado just prior to serving.

Per Serving: Calories: 459; Total fat: 36g; Total carbs: 9g; Fiber: 5g; Net carbs: 4g; Protein: 24g
Macros: 71% Fat; 21% Protein; 8% Carbs

Baked Chicken Alfredo with Spinach

CARDIO
Serves 6

Prep time: 5 mins
Cook time: 25 mins

This casserole provides energy for cardio workouts.

FOR THE SAUCE
8 tablespoons (1 stick) unsalted butter
4 garlic cloves, minced, or 2 teaspoons minced garlic
1 cup heavy cream
4 ounces full-fat cream cheese
1 cup freshly shredded Parmesan cheese
1 teaspoon kosher salt
½ teaspoon freshly ground black pepper

FOR THE CHICKEN
2 tablespoons extra-virgin olive oil
½ small yellow onion, minced
1 pound boneless skinless chicken thighs, cut into bite-size pieces
2 teaspoons dried oregano or basil (optional)
1 teaspoon kosher salt
16 ounces frozen spinach, thawed and drained
1 cup freshly shredded Parmesan cheese

1. Preheat the oven to 400°F.
2. **To make the sauce:** In a medium saucepan, melt the butter over low heat.
3. Add the garlic and sauté for 2 minutes, or until fragrant. Increase the heat to medium. Add the cream and cream cheese. Whisk until smooth. Add the Parmesan, salt, and pepper. Whisk until smooth. Remove from the heat.
4. **To make the chicken:** In a large skillet, heat the oil over medium-high heat.
5. Add the onion and sauté for 2 to 3 minutes, or until just tender. Add the chicken, oregano (if using), and salt. Sauté for 5 to 6 minutes, or until the chicken has cooked through. Add the spinach and sauce. Stir until well combined. Remove from the heat. Transfer the mixture to a 9-by-13-inch glass baking dish.
6. Top with the cheese. Transfer the baking dish to the oven and bake for 10 to 12 minutes, or until the sauce is bubbly and the cheese has melted. Remove from the oven. Serve warm.

Per Serving: Calories: 615; Total fat: 51g; Total carbs: 10g; Fiber: 2g; Net carbs: 8g; Protein: 28g
Macros: 75% Fat; 18% Protein; 7% Carbs

Greek Stuffed Chicken Breasts

STRENGTH TRAINING

Serves 4

Prep time: 20 mins
Cook time: 40 mins

This dish is a high-protein recovery meal perfect for post–strength training. Lean chicken breasts are stuffed with higher-fat feta cheese to keep them keto friendly.

8 tablespoons extra-virgin olive oil, divided
4 ounces frozen spinach, thawed and drained
4 ounces crumbled feta cheese
¼ cup chopped pitted Kalamata olives
2 teaspoons dried oregano
1 teaspoon kosher salt
1 teaspoon garlic powder
¼ teaspoon freshly ground black pepper
2 boneless skinless chicken breasts (about 1 pound total)
2 tablespoons balsamic vinegar

1. Preheat the oven to 375°F. Coat the bottom of a small baking dish with 1 tablespoon of oil.
2. In a medium bowl, combine the spinach, cheese, olives, oregano, salt, garlic powder, pepper, and 3 tablespoons of oil. Mix well.
3. Make a deep 2-inch-long incision along the length of each chicken breast to create a pocket. Using your knife or fingers, increase the size of the pocket without cutting through the chicken breast.
4. Stuff half of the spinach mixture into each breast. Place the breasts, cut-side up, in the prepared baking dish. Cover with aluminum foil.
5. Transfer the baking dish to the oven and bake for 30 to 40 minutes, or until the chicken has cooked through. Remove from the oven. Let rest, covered, for 10 minutes.
6. In a small bowl, whisk together the remaining olive oil and the vinegar.
7. To serve, cut each chicken breast in half widthwise and serve drizzled with 1½ tablespoons of the oil and vinegar mixture.

▶ **STORAGE TIP:** To prep ahead, wrap uncooked stuffed chicken breasts in plastic wrap or foil and refrigerate for up to 2 days before cooking.

Per Serving: Calories: 471; Total fat: 38g; Total carbs: 4g; Fiber: 0.5g; Net carbs: 3.5g; Protein: 28g
Macros: 73% Fat; 24% Protein; 3% Carbs

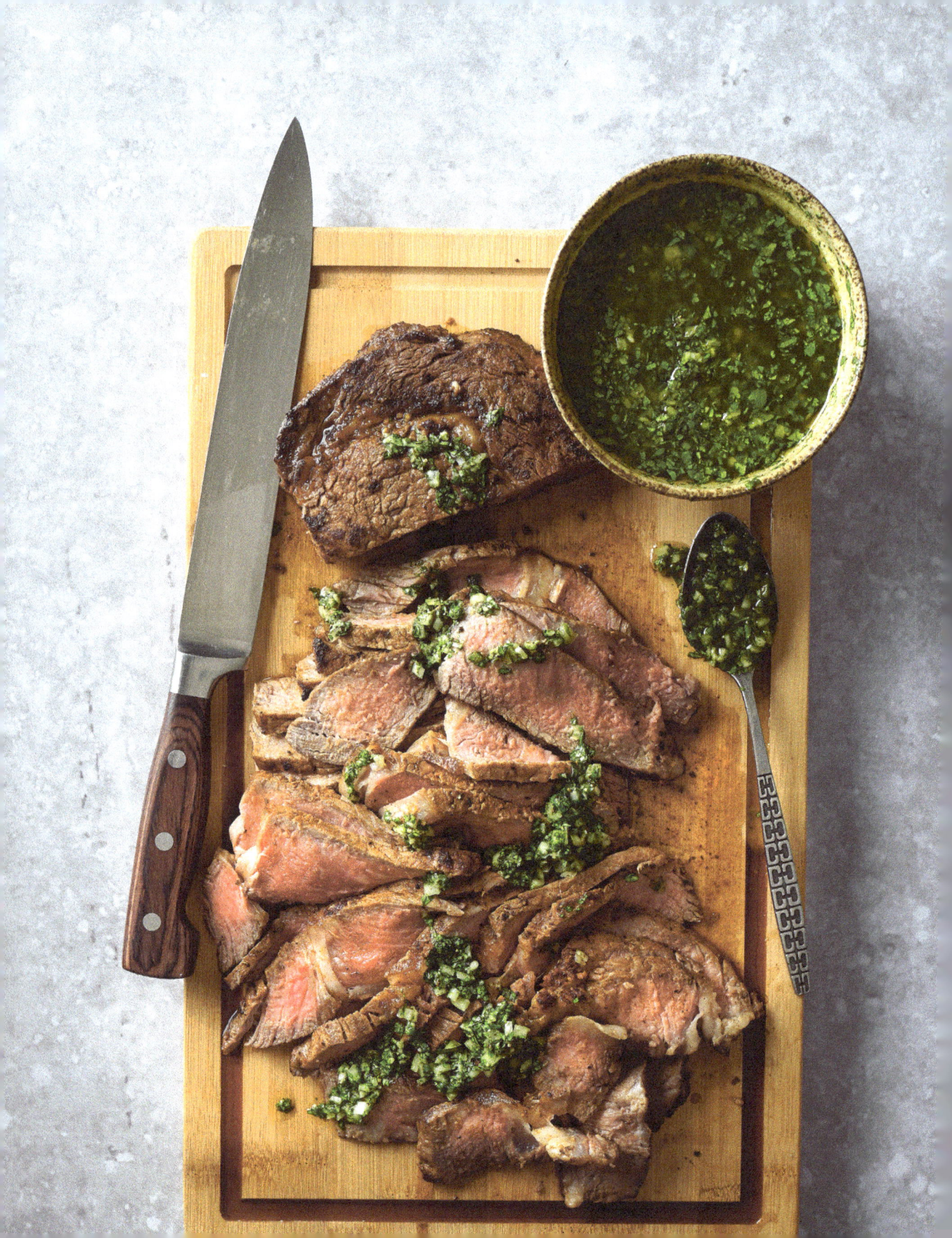

CHAPTER 7

Pork and Beef

Corn Bread Taco Pie 82

Chorizo and Cheese–Stuffed Poblanos 83

Easy Slow-Cooked Ribs 84

Thai-Inspired Ground Pork Lettuce Cups 85

Mozzarella-Stuffed Pork Loin 86

Shepherd's Pie 87

Eggplant Lasagna 89

Pesto Steak and Broccoli Foil Packs 91

Flank Steak with Easy Chimichurri Sauce 92

Braised Beef Short Ribs 93

Corn Bread Taco Pie

STRENGTH TRAINING

Serves 6

Prep time: 10 mins
Cook time: 40 mins

This higher carb keto recipe is great to have before heavy-lifting or sprint workouts.

- 4 tablespoons extra-virgin olive oil, divided
- 1 pound ground beef, preferably grass-fed
- 2 tablespoons taco seasoning
- 8 ounces full-fat cream cheese
- ½ cup no-sugar-added jarred salsa
- 1¼ cups almond flour
- ¼ cup cornmeal
- ½ teaspoon baking powder
- ½ teaspoon kosher salt
- 2 tablespoons unsalted butter, melted
- ¼ cup unsweetened almond milk
- 1 large egg, beaten
- ¼ cup frozen corn, thawed and chopped
- 3 cups shredded Mexican blend or cheddar cheese
- 1 cup sour cream

1. Preheat the oven to 375°F. Drizzle 2 tablespoons of oil into a 9-by-13-inch glass baking dish. Swirl to coat.
2. In a large skillet, heat the remaining olive oil over medium-high heat. Add the beef and sauté for 5 to 6 minutes, or until browned. Do not drain the fat.
3. Reduce the heat to medium. Add the taco seasoning and cream cheese. Stir until the cream cheese has melted.
4. Stir in the salsa. Remove from the heat.
5. In a large bowl, combine the almond flour, cornmeal, baking powder, and salt. Whisk until smooth.
6. Add the butter, almond milk, and egg. Whisk until combined. Stir in the corn. Pour the mixture into the prepared baking dish, spreading evenly. Top with the beef, then the shredded cheese.
7. Transfer the baking dish to the oven and bake for 20 to 25 minutes, or until the corn bread has cooked through. Remove from the oven. Let cool for 5 minutes before cutting. Garnish with the sour cream. Serve warm.

▶ **STORAGE TIP:** Store in the refrigerator for up to 4 days or in the freezer for up to 3 months.

Per Serving: Calories: 844; Total fat: 70g; Total carbs: 17g; Fiber: 3.5g; Net carbs: 13.5g; Protein: 36.5g
Macros: 75% Fat; 17% Protein; 8% Carbs

Chorizo and Cheese-Stuffed Poblanos

OVERALL FITNESS

Serves 4

Prep time: 20 mins
Cook time: 35 mins

Poblano peppers are mild in flavor and perfect for stuffing with cheesy sausage filling. If you can't find chorizo, substitute hot Italian pork sausage.

---

4 large poblano peppers
2 tablespoons olive oil
8 ounces fresh chorizo sausage

4 ounces full-fat cream cheese, at room temperature

4 ounces frozen spinach, thawed and drained
2 cups shredded Mexican cheese blend, divided

1. Preheat the oven to 400°F. Line a glass baking dish with aluminum foil.
2. Put the peppers in the prepared baking dish. Transfer the dish to the oven and roast for 15 to 20 minutes, or until the peppers are just soft. Remove from the oven, leaving the oven on. Let cool. Set aside the baking dish.
3. In a large skillet, heat the oil over medium-high heat.
4. Add the chorizo and cook for about 5 minutes, or until browned and the fat has rendered. Do not drain.
5. Reduce the heat to low. Add the cream cheese and spinach. Stir until well combined.
6. Add 1½ cups of shredded cheese and stir until melted and well blended. Remove from the heat.
7. Once cool, cut a slit in each pepper lengthwise, leaving about 1 inch on each end. Remove the seeds and membranes, leaving the rest intact.
8. Stuff each pepper with one-quarter of the chorizo and cheese mixture. Top each with 2 tablespoons of the remaining shredded cheese.
9. Place the peppers in the reserved baking dish. Transfer the baking dish to the oven and bake for 5 to 6 minutes, or until the cheese has melted. Remove from the oven. Serve the peppers whole.

▶ **STORAGE TIP:** Prep the filling in advance and store in the refrigerator for up to 4 days before stuffing and baking the peppers to serve.

Per Serving: Calories: 523; Total fat: 44g; Total carbs: 7g; Fiber: 2.5g; Net carbs: 4.5g; Protein: 25g
Macros: 76% Fat; 19% Protein; 5% Carbs

Easy Slow-Cooked Ribs

OVERALL FITNESS

Serves 4

Prep time: 10 mins
Cook time: 10 mins, plus 4 to 6 hrs inactive time

With very little hands-on prep time, these finger-licking ribs are a breeze to make. For an even easier prep, use bottled sugar-free barbecue sauce and add the splash of soy sauce for a unique twist.

- 1 (2½- to 3-pound) rack baby back pork ribs, cut into 3-rib segments
- 1½ cups no-sugar-added ketchup
- ¼ cup apple cider vinegar
- 2 tablespoons soy sauce
- 2 teaspoons granulated sugar-free sweetener (optional)
- 1 teaspoon garlic powder

1. Put the rib segments in a slow cooker. Alternatively, you can use a Dutch oven with the oven set to 250°F.
2. In a small bowl, whisk together the ketchup, vinegar, soy sauce, sweetener (if using), and garlic powder.
3. Pour 1 cup of the mixture over the ribs and toss to coat. Cook on low for 6 hours or in the oven for 4 hours. Turn off the slow cooker.
4. Preheat the oven to 500°F. Line a baking sheet with aluminum foil.
5. Put the ribs on the prepared baking sheet. Brush with the remaining sauce mixture.
6. Transfer the baking sheet to the oven and bake for 10 minutes, or until the ribs are browned and crispy on top. Remove from the oven. Serve hot.

▶ **STORAGE TIP:** The cooked ribs will store in the refrigerator for up to 4 days. Reheat in the oven to crisp and warm before serving.

Per Serving: Calories: 433; Total fat: 32g; Total carbs: 1g; Fiber: 0g; Net carbs: 1g; Protein: 35g
Macros: 67% Fat; 32% Protein; 1% Carbs

Thai-Inspired Ground Pork Lettuce Cups

OVERALL FITNESS

Serves 4

Prep time: 15 mins
Cook time: 15 mins

These lettuce cups have such fresh flavor you'll think you treated yourself to fancy take-out. I like Bibb lettuce leaves for their delicate texture and cup-like shape, but feel free to use romaine for more of a "boat" or iceberg for a crunchier texture.

- 2 tablespoons extra-virgin olive oil
- 1 pound mild ground pork sausage
- 2 tablespoons minced fresh ginger
- ½ cup chopped scallions, white and green parts
- 4 garlic cloves, minced
- 2 tablespoons fish sauce or tamari
- 1 cup chopped fresh cilantro or mint (or a combination of both)
- Grated zest and juice of 1 lime
- 2 tablespoons toasted sesame oil
- 8 Bibb lettuce leaves
- 2 ripe avocados, pitted, peeled, and sliced
- 1 lime, sliced (optional)
- Hot sauce, for serving (optional)

1. In a large skillet, heat the oil over medium heat.
2. Add the sausage and cook for 4 to 5 minutes, or until just browned and crumbly.
3. Add the ginger and cook for 2 minutes, or until fragrant.
4. Add the scallions, garlic, and fish sauce. Sauté for 2 to 3 minutes, or until the pork has cooked through and the scallions are tender. Remove from the heat.
5. Stir in the cilantro, lime zest, lime juice, and sesame oil.
6. To serve, place the meat mixture in each lettuce cup and top with the avocado.
7. Garnish with lime (if using) and hot sauce (if using).

▶ **STORAGE TIP:** Prep the pork mixture in advance and store it in the refrigerator for up to 4 days before reheating to assemble lettuce cups.

Per Serving: Calories: 524; Total fat: 45g; Total carbs: 10g; Fiber: 5.5g; Net carbs: 4.5g; Protein: 19g
Macros: 77% Fat; 15% Protein; 8% Carbs

Mozzarella-Stuffed Pork Loin

OVERALL FITNESS
Serves 12

Prep time: 25 mins
Cook time: 30 mins

This beautifully presented dish is great for entertaining. It uses two packs of pork tenderloin, plenty for leftovers or for feeding a crowd.

- 2 (1- to 1½-pound) pork tenderloins
- 4 tablespoons olive oil, divided
- 2 cups shredded mozzarella cheese
- 4 ounces frozen spinach, thawed and drained
- 8 ounces full-fat cream cheese, at room temperature
- 1 cup no-sugar-added marinara sauce
- 1 teaspoon kosher salt
- 1 teaspoon garlic powder
- ¼ teaspoon freshly ground black pepper

1. Preheat the oven to 375°F.
2. Without cutting through to the other side, make a deep slit lengthwise along each tenderloin, leaving about 2 inches on each end to create a pocket. Using your fingers, carefully increase the size of the pocket.
3. Using your hands, spread 2 tablespoons of oil over each tenderloin, coating the inside of the pocket and the outside of each tenderloin. Transfer to a 9-by-13-inch glass baking dish.
4. In a medium bowl, combine the mozzarella cheese, spinach, cream cheese, marinara sauce, salt, garlic powder, and pepper. Stir until well combined.
5. Stuff half of the mixture into each tenderloin and, using your hands, press the opening together to seal. Cover the tenderloins with aluminum foil.
6. Transfer the baking dish to the oven and bake for 20 to 25 minutes (depending on the size of the tenderloins), or until cooked through.
7. Remove the foil and bake for 5 minutes to brown the outsides. Remove from the oven. Let sit for 10 minutes before slicing. Serve warm.

▶ **STORAGE TIP:** The stuffed pork can be frozen raw. If feeding only a few people, prepare the full recipe and then cook one loin, freezing the other.

Per Serving: Calories: 306; Total fat: 22g; Total carbs: 3g; Fiber: 0.5g; Net carbs: 2.5g; Protein: 24g
Macros: 65% Fat; 31% Protein; 4% Carbs

Shepherd's Pie

CARDIO
Serves 8

Prep time: 15 mins
Cook time: 1 hr

With high fat ratios, this is a great dish for sustained energy during longer cardio workouts. Frozen cauliflower makes it easy to prep this satisfying meal.

- 2 cups frozen cauliflower florets, thawed
- ½ cup heavy cream
- 4 tablespoons (½ stick) unsalted butter
- 1 cup shredded cheddar cheese
- 2 teaspoons kosher salt, divided
- 2 teaspoons dried thyme or oregano, divided
- ¼ teaspoon freshly ground black pepper
- 2 tablespoons extra-virgin olive oil
- 1 pound ground beef, preferably grass-fed
- 4 ounces mushrooms, sliced
- 1 cup chopped cabbage
- ½ yellow onion, diced
- 1 carrot, diced
- 2 celery stalks, diced
- 4 garlic cloves, minced
- 1 (15-ounce) can tomato puree
- 8 ounces full-fat cream cheese, at room temperature

1. Preheat the oven to 375°F.
2. In a microwave-safe bowl, combine the cauliflower, cream, and butter. Cover with a paper towel and microwave for 60 to 90 seconds, or until the cauliflower is tender. Stir in the cheddar cheese, 1 teaspoon of salt, 1 teaspoon of thyme, and the pepper. Using an immersion blender or hand mixer, puree until smooth.
3. In a large saucepan or skillet, heat the oil over medium-high heat.
4. Add the beef and sauté, breaking it apart with a spoon, for 5 minutes. Add the mushrooms, cabbage, onion, carrot, and celery. Sauté for 5 to 6 minutes, or until the beef has browned.
5. Add the garlic, remaining 1 teaspoon of salt, and remaining 1 teaspoon of thyme. Sauté for 30 seconds. Stir in the tomato puree and cream cheese. Bring to a simmer.
6. Reduce the heat to low. Simmer, stirring occasionally, for 8 to 10 minutes, or until the vegetables are tender. Remove from the heat. Transfer to an 8-by-8-inch glass baking dish.

CONTINUED ➡

Shepherd's Pie CONTINUED

7. Spread the cauliflower mixture on top. Transfer the baking dish to the oven and bake for 25 to 30 minutes, or until golden. Remove from the oven. Let rest for 5 minutes. Serve warm.

▶ **STORAGE TIP:** Double the recipe and freeze the second pie for later. Thaw in the refrigerator overnight and bake at 375°F for 20 to 25 minutes.

Per Serving: Calories: 429; Total fat: 35g; Total carbs: 11.5g; Fiber: 2.5g; Net carbs: 9g; Protein: 17g
Macros: 73% Fat; 16% Protein; 11% Carbs

Eggplant Lasagna

OVERALL FITNESS
Serves 8

Prep time: 15 mins
Cook time: 1 hr

This version of the comfort food favorite is so full of flavor you won't miss the pasta!

- 10 tablespoons extra-virgin olive oil, divided
- 2 small eggplants, cut lengthwise into ¼-inch-thick slices
- 1 teaspoon kosher salt
- 1 pound ground beef, preferably grass-fed
- 2 cups whole-milk ricotta cheese
- 2 teaspoons dried basil or oregano
- 1 teaspoon garlic powder
- 1 (24-ounce) jar no-sugar-added marinara sauce
- 2 cups shredded mozzarella cheese

1. Preheat the oven to 425°F. Line 2 baking sheets with parchment paper. Drizzle each with 2 tablespoons of oil, spreading evenly.
2. Put the eggplants on the prepared baking sheets. Sprinkle with the salt.
3. Transfer the baking sheets to the oven and bake for 10 to 12 minutes, or until the eggplants have softened but are not mushy. Remove from the oven. Let cool slightly.
4. Reduce the oven temperature to 375°F.
5. While the eggplants roast, in a large skillet, heat 2 tablespoons of oil over medium-high heat.
6. Add the beef and cook for about 5 minutes, or until browned. Remove from the heat. Transfer to a medium bowl.
7. Add the ricotta cheese, basil, and garlic powder. Stir to combine.
8. In another bowl, mix together the marinara sauce and remaining 4 tablespoons of oil.
9. Spoon one-third of the marinara into a 9-by-13-inch glass baking dish and spread evenly.
10. Place a layer of eggplant slices to cover the sauce, then spread one-third of the beef and ricotta mixture evenly.
11. Sprinkle one-third of the mozzarella cheese on top. Repeat with 2 more layers of each. Cover the baking dish with aluminum foil.

CONTINUED ➡

Eggplant Lasagna CONTINUED

12. Transfer the baking dish to the oven and bake for 30 minutes, or until the cheese has melted.

13. Remove the foil. Bake for 5 to 8 minutes, or until the lasagna has browned. Remove from the oven. Let rest for 5 minutes before slicing. Serve warm.

▶ **STORAGE TIP:** This lasagna freezes really well, so consider making two and freezing the second for a quick meal later.

Per Serving: Calories: 528; Total fat: 40g; Total carbs: 17g; Fiber: 4g; Net carbs: 13g; Protein: 25g
Macros: 68% Fat; 19% Protein; 13% Carbs

Pesto Steak and Broccoli Foil Packs

OVERALL FITNESS

Serves 4

Prep time: 20 mins
Cook time: 15 mins

These little ready-to-grill foil packs are easy to prep in advance for a high-fat, low-carb, complete-protein meal. If you don't have a grill, bake in the oven at 400°F for 10 to 12 minutes.

---

1 (12-ounce) steamable bag broccoli florets or 2 cups broccoli florets

2 tablespoons olive oil
1 pound flank steak, cut into bite-size chunks

1 (4-ounce) jar basil pesto

1. Preheat the grill on medium-high heat.
2. Steam the broccoli until lightly tender. Or if using fresh, place the florets in a microwave-safe bowl, add ¼ cup of water, cover, and microwave on high for 2 to 3 minutes, or until tender. Drain.
3. In a large skillet, heat the oil over medium-high heat.
4. Add the steak and brown on all sides for about 2 minutes per side. Do not cook all the way through. Remove from the heat.
5. Add the steamed broccoli and pesto. Toss to coat well.
6. Lay 4 (8-inch) squares of aluminum foil on the counter. Place one-quarter of the steak mixture in the middle of each piece of foil. Cover each with a second foil square and fold the foil up to about 1 inch from the mixture on each side. Fold in each corner once to secure and seal the foil packs.
7. Place the foil packs in a single layer on the hot grill and grill for 4 to 6 minutes, or until the steak has cooked through and the broccoli is fork tender. Remove from the heat.

▶ **STORAGE TIP:** These freeze beautifully. To reheat, simply thaw completely before cooking per the recipe.

Per Serving: Calories: 375; Total fat: 27g; Total carbs: 5g; Fiber: 1g; Net carbs: 4g; Protein: 28g
Macros: 65% Fat; 30% Protein; 5% Carbs

Flank Steak with Easy Chimichurri Sauce

OVERALL FITNESS

Serves 4

Prep time: 10 mins
Cook time: 20 mins

This is an intensely flavorful, high-protein dish that comes together really quickly. Serve with a side of roasted veggies or over a bed of mixed greens, using extra chimichurri as dressing.

- 1 pound flank steak
- 10 tablespoons olive oil, divided
- 1 teaspoon kosher salt
- ½ teaspoon freshly ground black pepper
- 1 cup packed fresh cilantro or mint
- 4 garlic cloves, peeled
- Grated zest and juice of 1 orange
- 2 tablespoons tamari
- 1 teaspoon red pepper flakes (optional)

1. Heat the grill on medium-high heat, or preheat the oven to 450°F.
2. Rub the steak with 2 tablespoons of oil. Sprinkle with the salt and black pepper. Let sit at room temperature while you make the chimichurri.
3. To make the chimichurri, in a food processor, combine the cilantro, garlic, orange zest, orange juice, tamari, and red pepper flakes (if using). Pulse until a finely chopped paste forms. With the processor running, stream in the remaining 8 tablespoons of oil and process until well combined.
4. Put the steak on the grill and cook for 6 to 8 minutes per side, or to your desired doneness. If using an oven, heat an oven-safe skillet (preferably cast-iron) over high heat. Sear the steak for 1 to 2 minutes per side, remove from the heat, and transfer to the oven to roast for 8 to 10 minutes, or until it reaches your desired doneness. Remove from the oven. Let rest for 5 minutes before slicing.
5. Serve the steak drizzled with the chimichurri.

▶ **STORAGE TIP:** Chimichurri is wonderful mixed with scrambled eggs or as a sauce for grilled fish or chicken. This sauce will last in a sealed container for up to 2 weeks.

Per Serving: Calories: 494; Total fat: 41g; Total carbs: 3.5g; Fiber: 0g; Net carbs: 3.5g; Protein: 27g
Macros: 75% Fat; 22% Protein; 3% Carbs

Braised Beef Short Ribs

CARDIO
Serves 4

Prep time: 10 mins
Cook time: 2 hrs

This rich high-fat meal provides sustained energy for longer cardio workouts. Don't skimp on the cooking time; searing the meat locks in flavor, and slow braising keeps the meat moist and tender.

1½ pounds boneless beef short ribs (if using bone-in, use 3½ pounds)
1 teaspoon kosher salt
¼ teaspoon freshly ground black pepper
¼ cup extra-virgin olive oil
1 cup dry red wine, such as cabernet sauvignon or merlot
2 to 3 cups beef broth
1 teaspoon garlic powder
1 teaspoon dried thyme or rosemary

1. Preheat the oven to 350°F.
2. Season the short ribs with the salt and pepper.
3. In a Dutch oven or deep oven-safe skillet, heat the oil over medium-high heat.
4. When the oil is very hot, add the short ribs and brown for 2 to 3 minutes per side, or until dark in color. Remove the short ribs from the oil and keep warm.
5. To the rendered fat and oil in the Dutch oven, add the wine, 2 cups of broth, the garlic powder, and thyme. Whisk together and bring to a boil.
6. Reduce the heat to low. Simmer for about 10 minutes, or until the liquid has reduced to 2 cups.
7. Return the short ribs to the liquid and add enough broth so that the liquid covers the meat halfway. Cover with the lid. Remove from the heat.
8. Transfer the pot to the oven and braise for 1½ to 2 hours, or until the meat is very tender. Remove from the oven. Let sit covered for 10 minutes before serving. Serve the beef warm, drizzled with the cooking liquid.

▶ **STORAGE TIP:** Cooked ribs will store in the refrigerator for up to 4 days.

Per Serving: Calories: 398; Total fat: 27g; Total carbs: 3g; Fiber: 0g; Net carbs: 3g; Protein: 25g
Macros: 61% Fat; 25% Protein; 3% Carbs

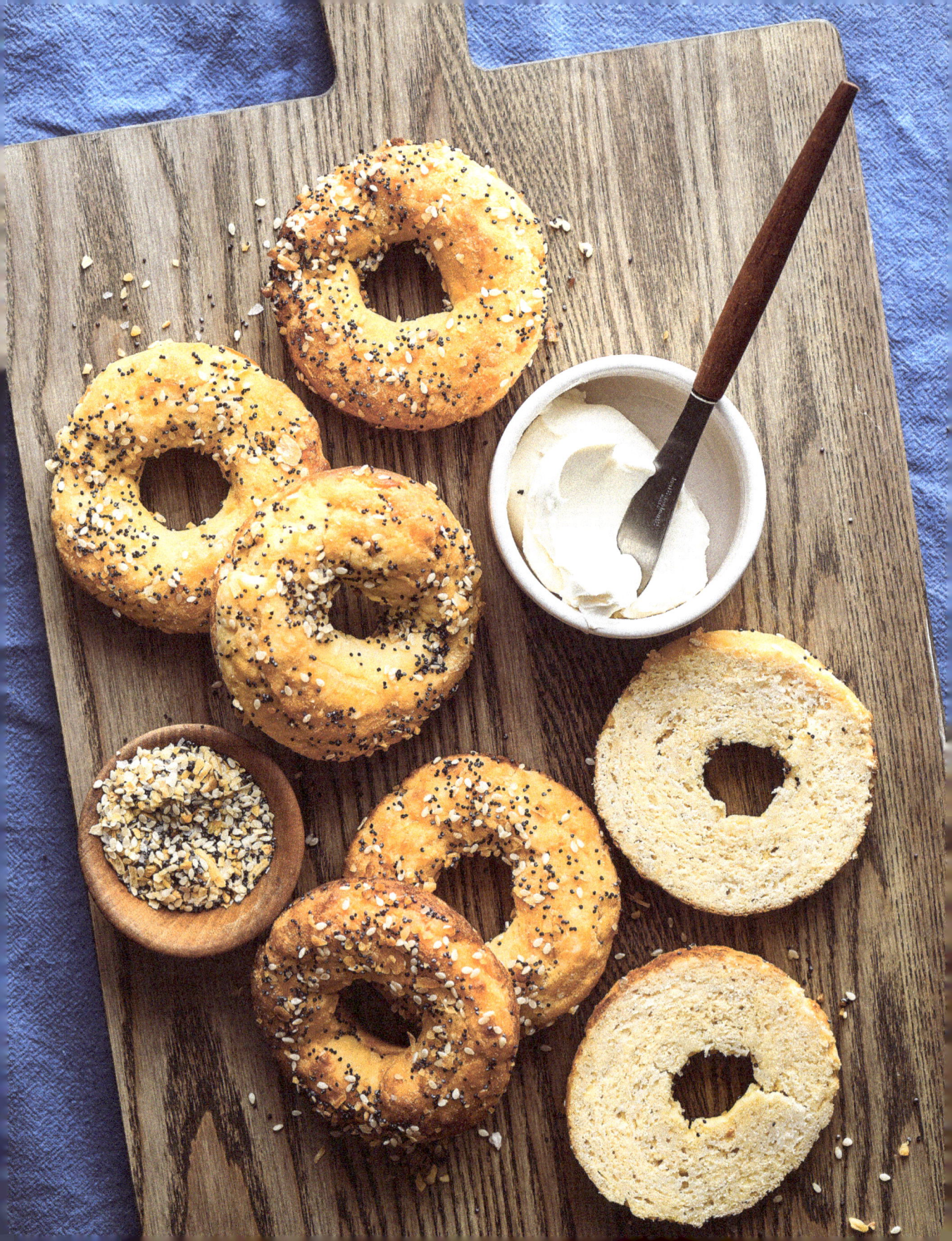

CHAPTER 8

Snacks and Staples

Lemon-Tahini Sauce 96

Molly's Flavor-Filled Mayo 97

Coconut–Nut Butter Power Balls 98

90-Second Keto Dinner Roll 99

Keto Bagels 100

Creamy Avocado Dressing 101

Crave-Worthy Caesar Dressing 102

Cashew Hummus 103

Lemon-Tahini Sauce

OVERALL FITNESS

Makes 1 cup

Prep time: 10 mins

This creamy, dairy-free sauce is perfect for dressing salads. It is also delicious as a dipping sauce for grilled meats or for tossing with roasted vegetables, like Brussels sprouts. Tahini is a ground sesame seed paste and is found in most grocery stores, either in the international foods aisle or with the other nut and seed butters.

¼ cup extra-virgin olive oil

¼ cup tahini

¼ cup freshly squeezed lemon juice (from about 2 large lemons)

3 tablespoons tamari

2 garlic cloves, minced, or 2 teaspoons garlic powder

In a small bowl or glass, whisk together the oil, tahini, lemon juice, tamari, and garlic until very smooth. Refrigerate until ready to use.

▶ **STORAGE TIP:** This sauce will store in the refrigerator for up to 6 days. Separation is natural; whisk to combine before serving.

Per Serving (2 tablespoons): Calories: 110; Total fat: 10g; Total carbs: 3g; Fiber: 0.5g; Net carbs: 2.5g; Protein: 2g
Macros: 82% Fat; 7% Protein; 11% Carbs

Molly's Flavor-Filled Mayo

OVERALL FITNESS

Makes 1 cup

Prep time: 5 mins

This mayonnaise-based sauce is so easy to whip up and is a flavorful way to add healthy energizing fat to just about everything from meats or fish to vegetables or eggs. Play with the seasonings to your preference. Add a dash of hot sauce or cayenne pepper for a spicier sauce.

½ cup no-sugar-added ketchup
½ cup mayonnaise
1 teaspoon garlic powder
1 teaspoon onion powder
¼ teaspoon paprika
1 teaspoon kosher salt

In a small bowl, whisk together the ketchup, mayonnaise, garlic powder, onion powder, paprika, and salt until smooth and creamy. Refrigerate until ready to use.

▶ **STORAGE TIP:** This sauce will store covered tightly in the refrigerator for up to 2 weeks.

Per Serving (2 tablespoons): Calories: 105; Total fat: 10g; Total carbs: 2.5g; Fiber: 0g; Net carbs: 2.5g; Protein: 1g
Macros: 86% Fat; 4% Protein; 10% Carbs

Coconut-Nut Butter Power Balls

STRENGTH TRAINING

Makes 1 dozen

Prep time: 20 mins, plus 1 hr to chill

These power balls are similar to popular keto fat bombs in consistency and convenience, but they have extra protein for post-workout recovery. Grab two or three for a quick and easy on-the-go breakfast after a morning workout, or use them as a protein-dense snack between meals. I prefer collagen peptides to other protein powders for the added benefit of gut health and tissue repair.

- 1 cup unsweetened peanut or almond butter, stirred well
- ½ cup unflavored collagen peptides or other protein powder
- ¼ cup almond or coconut flour
- ¼ cup granulated sugar-free sweetener, such as Swerve
- ¼ cup unsweetened coconut flakes
- 2 tablespoons chia seeds
- 1 teaspoon ground cinnamon

1. In a large bowl, combine the peanut butter, collagen peptides, almond flour, sweetener, coconut flakes, chia seeds, and cinnamon. Using your hands, mix everything together and shape into 12 (1-inch) balls. The mixture will be sticky.

2. Place the balls in a single layer on a baking sheet or in a large container. Refrigerate for at least 1 hour before serving.

▶ **STORAGE TIP:** Store these power balls in an airtight container in the refrigerator for up to 1 week or in the freezer for up to 3 months.

Per Serving (2 power balls): Calories: 400; Total fat: 28g; Total carbs: 16g; Fiber: 5g; Net carbs: 7g; Protein: 21g
Macros: 63% Fat; 21% Protein; 16% Carbs

90-Second Keto Dinner Roll

STRENGTH TRAINING

Serves 1

Prep time: 5 mins
Cook time: 90 seconds

High in energy-producing healthy fats, this is a great pre-endurance workout snack or can be part of a larger meal. The bread naturally has protein from the almond flour and egg, so spread some peanut butter or cream cheese on it for an even higher-fat snack or light meal.

- 2 tablespoons almond flour
- 1 tablespoon extra-virgin olive oil
- 1 large egg
- ¼ teaspoon baking powder
- ¼ teaspoon kosher salt

1. In a microwave-safe ramekin or wide mug or glass, combine the almond flour, oil, egg, baking powder, and salt. Using a fork, mix well. Microwave on high power for 90 seconds. Carefully remove from the microwave (the edges will be hot).

2. Slide a knife around the edges of the ramekin and flip to remove the bread. Eat whole as a roll, or slice in half with a serrated knife to make a sandwich.

▶ **STORAGE TIP:** Cooked rolls will store covered in the refrigerator for 1 or 2 days. Do not freeze.

Per Serving (1 dinner roll): Calories: 225; Total fat: 21g; Total carbs: 1g; Fiber: 0.5g; Net carbs: 0.5g; Protein: 8g
Macros: 84% Fat; 14% Protein; 2% Carbs

Keto Bagels

OVERALL FITNESS
Makes 6 bagels

Prep time: 15 mins
Cook time: 15 mins

Who doesn't love a bagel sandwich? With this easy-to-make variety, you can be keto fit and eat your bagels, too! Top with poppy seeds, sesame seeds, or everything seasoning for a more authentic bagel shop experience.

| 2½ cups shredded mozzarella cheese | 2 ounces full-fat cream cheese, at room temperature
1½ cups almond flour | 2 large eggs, beaten
1 tablespoon baking powder
½ teaspoon kosher salt |

1. Preheat the oven to 400°F. Line a baking sheet with parchment paper.
2. In a large microwave-safe bowl, combine the mozzarella cheese and cream cheese. Microwave on high for 90 seconds. Stir and microwave on high for another 30 seconds, or until fully melted. Stir well to combine.
3. Add the almond flour, eggs, baking powder, and salt. Using your hands, combine the mixture well, kneading until a dough comes together. The mixture will be sticky.
4. Divide the dough into 6 equal balls. Roll each into a long (8-inch) cylinder. Form into a circle to make a bagel shape, pressing the ends together to seal. Transfer to the prepared baking sheet.
5. Transfer the baking sheet to the oven and bake for 12 to 14 minutes, or until the bagels are golden brown. Remove from the oven.

▶ **STORAGE TIP:** Store leftover bagels in a sealed container in the refrigerator for up to 1 week or in the freezer for up to 3 months. Thaw, slice, and toast before serving for the best texture.

Per Serving (1 bagel): Calories: 360; Total fat: 24g; Total carbs: 14g; Fiber: 2g; Net carbs: 12g; Protein: 22g
Macros: 60% Fat; 24% Protein; 16% Carbs

Creamy Avocado Dressing

CARDIO

Makes 1½ cups

Prep time: 10 mins

Vegan and full of heart-healthy and energy-sustaining fats, this creamy dressing is a wonderful ranch alternative on Cobb salads or drizzled over grilled meats, fish, or vegetables.

2 very ripe avocados, pitted and peeled
¼ cup freshly squeezed lime juice (from about 4 limes)
1 teaspoon garlic powder
1 teaspoon kosher salt
¼ teaspoon freshly ground black pepper
½ cup extra-virgin olive oil

1. Put the avocados, lime juice, garlic powder, salt, and pepper in a blender. Blend until smooth.

2. With the blender running, stream in the oil until the mixture is creamy and well blended. If the mixture seems too thick, blend in warm water 1 tablespoon at a time.

▶ **STORAGE TIP:** Store this dressing in an airtight container in the refrigerator for up to 1 week.

Per Serving (2 tablespoons): Calories: 120; Total fat: 12g; Total carbs: 2g; Fiber: 1.5g; Net carbs: 0.5g; Protein: 1g
Macros: 90% Fat; 3% Protein; 7% Carbs

Crave-Worthy Caesar Dressing

OVERALL FITNESS

Makes about 1½ cups

Prep time: 10 mins

A go-to homemade dressing for adding flavorful and healthy fats to salads is key to keeping the keto-fit meal plan simple and tasty. Don't be tempted to omit the anchovy paste, since it is what gives this dressing that wonderful umami flavor. I love the unique flavor the dried tarragon brings to this dressing, but feel free to leave it out if you don't have any on hand.

1 cup mayonnaise
2 tablespoons freshly squeezed lemon juice
1 tablespoon Dijon mustard
1 tablespoon Worcestershire sauce
2 teaspoons anchovy paste
1 teaspoon garlic powder
1 teaspoon dried tarragon (optional)
¼ teaspoon kosher salt, plus more as needed
¼ teaspoon freshly ground black pepper

In a medium bowl or glass jar, whisk together the mayonnaise, lemon juice, mustard, Worcestershire sauce, anchovy paste, garlic powder, tarragon (if using), salt, and pepper until well combined, smooth, and creamy. Taste and adjust the salt to your liking.

▶ **STORAGE TIP:** This dressing will store in an airtight container in the refrigerator for up to 2 weeks.

Per Serving (2 tablespoons): Calories: 130; Total fat: 14g; Total carbs: 1g; Fiber: 0g; Net carbs: 1g; Protein: 0g
Macros: 97% Fat; 0% Protein; 3% Carbs

Cashew Hummus

OVERALL FITNESS

Makes 1 cup

Prep time: 5 mins, plus 8 hrs to soak

Hummus is a wonderful, convenient snack. But traditional hummus, high in carbohydrates, doesn't fit into a ketogenic diet. This version is not only keto-friendly, but full of anti-inflammatory ingredients to help with recovery and satiety post-workout. The cashews will need to be soaked in water overnight, so make sure to plan the added soaking time into your meal prep.

---

1 cup raw cashews
3 tablespoons tahini
2 garlic cloves, peeled
1 tablespoon freshly squeezed lemon juice
1 teaspoon kosher salt
¼ teaspoon freshly ground black pepper
¼ cup extra-virgin olive oil

1. Put the cashews in a medium bowl and cover with cold water. Cover the bowl and refrigerate overnight or up to 24 hours.
2. Drain the cashews. Transfer to a food processor.
3. Add the tahini and garlic. Process until smooth.
4. Add the lemon juice, salt, and pepper. Pulse until well combined.
5. With the processor running, stream in the oil and process until very smooth and creamy.

▶ **STORAGE TIP:** This hummus will store in a sealed container in the refrigerator for up to 4 days.

Per Serving (2 tablespoons): Calories: 176; Total fat: 16g; Total carbs: 5g; Fiber: 1g; Net carbs: 4g; Protein: 3g
Macros: 82% Fat; 7% Protein; 11% Carbs

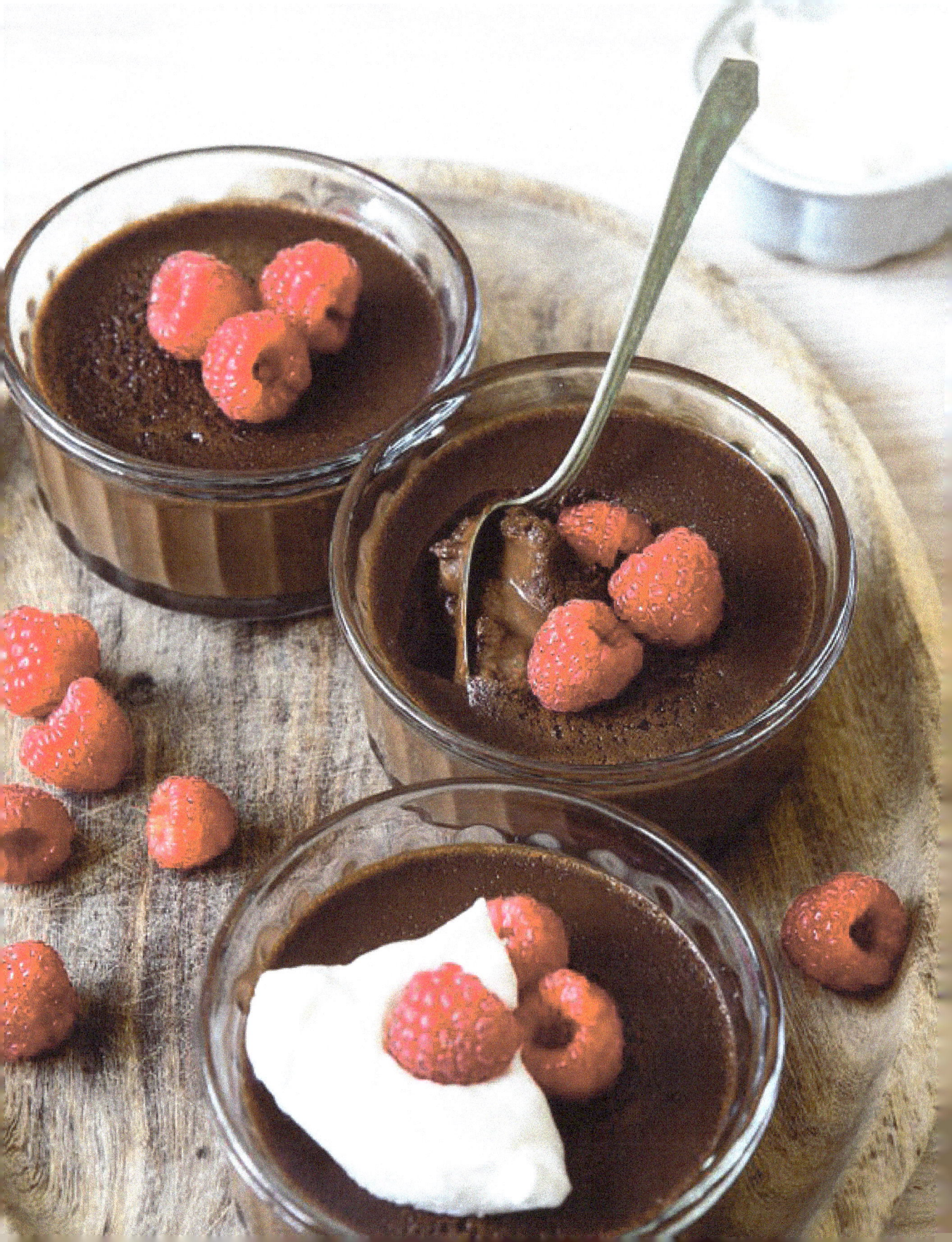

CHAPTER 9

Desserts

Cherry, Chocolate, and Chia Pudding 106

Dark Chocolate Mousse 107

Cookie Dough Fat Bombs 108

Cinnamon Streusel Cupcakes 109

Lemon-Poppy Seed Pound Cake 110

Chocolate-Peanut Butter Cups 111

Lime-Coconut Cream Pops 112

Cherry, Chocolate, and Chia Pudding

OVERALL FITNESS
Serves 4

Prep time: 10 mins, plus 6 hrs to chill

The powerful antioxidants in dark cherries help reduce inflammation, making them wonderful for recovery after a strenuous workout. The fruit gives this just enough sweetness, but feel free to add sugar-free sweetener to taste, if you prefer.

---

1 cup frozen dark red cherries, thawed with their juices

1 cup unsweetened almond milk

½ cup heavy cream

1 teaspoon vanilla extract

½ cup chia seeds

1 tablespoon unsweetened cocoa powder

1. Put the cherries in a blender or food processor and blend until smooth. Alternatively, chop them well for a coarser texture.
2. In a medium bowl, whisk together the almond milk, cream, and vanilla.
3. Add the chia seeds and cocoa powder. Whisk until well combined.
4. Stir in the blended cherries and their juices.
5. Divide the mixture among 4 ramekins or small jars. Cover and refrigerate for at least 6 hours. Serve cold.

▶ **STORAGE TIP:** This pudding will store covered in the refrigerator for up to 1 week.

Per Serving: Calories: 246; Total fat: 18g; Total carbs: 16g; Fiber: 8.5g; Net carbs: 7.5g; Protein: 5g
Macros: 66% Fat; 8% Protein; 26% Carbs

Dark Chocolate Mousse

OVERALL FITNESS

Serves 4

Prep time: 15 mins

Light and fluffy, this mousse couldn't be easier to make! Make sure to use chilled cream, not the shelf-stable variety. For intense dark-chocolate flavor, I like using Hershey's Special Dark cocoa powder, but any unsweetened cocoa powder will do.

---

1 cup heavy cream, chilled
1 teaspoon vanilla extract

¼ cup unsweetened cocoa powder
¼ cup powdered sugar-free sweetener, such as Swerve

¼ cup sugar-free mini chocolate chips

1. In a large bowl, combine the cream and vanilla. Using a hand mixer, beat on high speed for 2 to 3 minutes, or until stiff peaks form, being careful not to overbeat. Turn off the mixer. (You can also use a whisk; it will take you closer to 5 to 6 minutes of beating, but it is a great arm workout!)

2. Sift together the cocoa powder and sweetener into a medium bowl. Add to the whipped cream.

3. Add the chocolate chips and whisk together until smooth. Serve immediately, or chill for up to 1 hour.

▶ **STORAGE TIP:** For a fluffy texture, this dessert is best served right away, but it will keep covered in the refrigerator for up to 2 days.

Per Serving: Calories: 342; Total fat: 26g; Total carbs: 24g; Fiber: 2g; Net carbs: 7g; Protein: 3g
Macros: 68% Fat; 4% Protein; 28% Carbs

Cookie Dough Fat Bombs

CARDIO

Makes 8 fat bombs

Prep time: 15 mins, plus 30 mins to chill

The best part about making cookies is eating the dough. With these ketone-making little treats, you'll feel just as indulgent. Adjust the sweetener to your taste. Chopped nuts, such as walnuts or pecans, are also delicious additions to these bombs if you are craving even more flavor and texture.

- 8 tablespoons (1 stick) unsalted butter, at room temperature
- ¼ cup granulated sugar-free sweetener, such as Swerve
- 1 teaspoon vanilla extract
- 1½ cups almond flour
- ⅓ cup sugar-free mini chocolate chips

1. In a large bowl, combine the butter, sweetener, and vanilla. Using an electric mixer, mix on medium speed for 1 to 2 minutes, or until creamy and smooth. Turn off the mixer.
2. Add the almond flour and stir until well incorporated.
3. Stir in the chocolate chips and refrigerate the mixture for at least 30 minutes to allow it to harden slightly.
4. Using your hands, form the mixture into 8 balls. Place in a single layer in a large container.

▶ **STORAGE TIP:** These fat bombs will store sealed in the refrigerator for up to 1 week or in the freezer for up to 2 months.

Per Serving (1 fat bomb): Calories: 287; Total fat: 23g; Total carbs: 15g; Fiber: 3g; Net carbs: 3g; Protein: 5g
Macros: 72% Fat; 7% Protein; 21% Carbs

Cinnamon Streusel Cupcakes

OVERALL FITNESS
Makes 6 cupcakes

Prep time: 20 mins
Cook time: 20 mins

The cinnamon streusel on top of these cupcakes makes them perfect as a dessert or as an indulgent breakfast treat. These cupcakes are best fresh right out of the oven.

1¼ cups almond flour, divided
2 tablespoons granulated sugar-free sweetener, such as Swerve, plus ¼ cup
2 tablespoons unsalted butter, cut into small pieces
2 teaspoons ground cinnamon, divided
1 large egg
½ cup coconut oil, melted
1 teaspoon vanilla extract
1 teaspoon baking powder

1. Preheat the oven to 350°F. Line a 6-cup muffin tin with paper liners.
2. Put ¼ cup of almond flour, 2 tablespoons of sweetener, the butter, and 1 teaspoon of cinnamon in a small bowl. Using a fork or your fingers, combine until crumbly.
3. To make the batter, in a large bowl, whisk together the egg and remaining ¼ cup of sweetener.
4. Add the oil, vanilla, and remaining 1 teaspoon of cinnamon. Whisk until smooth.
5. To the large bowl, add the remaining 1 cup of almond flour and the baking powder. Stir until just combined.
6. Divide the batter evenly into the prepared muffin cups.
7. Top with 1 tablespoon of the cinnamon mixture, pressing lightly so it adheres to the batter.
8. Transfer the muffin tin to the oven and bake for 18 to 20 minutes, or until a toothpick inserted into the cupcake center comes out clean. Remove from the oven. Let cool for 5 minutes in the tin before serving warm.

▶ **STORAGE TIP:** Store these cupcakes in a sealed container in the refrigerator for up to 4 days or in the freezer for up to 2 months. Reheat in the microwave before serving.

Per Serving (1 cupcake): Calories: 366; Total fat: 32g; Total carbs: 15g; Fiber: 3g; Net carbs: 4.5g; Protein: 5g
Macros: 79% Fat; 5% Protein; 16% Carbs

Lemon-Poppy Seed Pound Cake

CARDIO
Serves 8

Prep time: 10 mins
Cook time: 45 mins

This sweet treat is a client favorite and full of energizing keto fats. The xanthan gum gives this cake structure and helps avoid a crumbly consistency. Serve with fresh blueberries when they are in season for a wonderful presentation.

- 13 tablespoons unsalted butter, melted, divided
- ½ cup sour cream
- ½ cup granulated sugar-free sweetener, such as Swerve
- 3 large eggs
- 1 teaspoon vanilla extract
- Grated zest of 2 lemons
- 1¾ cups almond flour
- 1½ teaspoons baking powder
- 1½ teaspoons poppy seeds
- 1 teaspoon xanthan gum

1. Preheat the oven to 350°F. Grease the bottom and sides of an 8-by-4-inch loaf pan with 1 tablespoon of butter.

2. In a large bowl, combine the remaining 12 tablespoons of butter, the sour cream, sweetener, eggs, vanilla, and lemon zest. Whisk until smooth and creamy.

3. Add the almond flour, baking powder, poppy seeds, and xanthan gum. Whisk until just blended. Pour the mixture into the prepared loaf pan.

4. Transfer the loaf pan to the oven and bake for 40 to 45 minutes, or until the top is very golden brown. Remove from the oven. Let cool for 15 minutes before removing the cake from the loaf pan. Cut into 8 slices to serve.

▶ **STORAGE TIP:** Store in the freezer for quick and easy single-serve portions. Slice the cake, wrap individual servings in aluminum foil, and store in a freezer-safe bag for up to 3 months.

Per Serving (1 slice): Calories: 402; Total fat: 34g; Total carbs: 17g; Fiber: 3g; Net carbs: 5.5g; Protein: 7g
Macros: 76% Fat; 7% Protein; 17% Carbs

Chocolate–Peanut Butter Cups

CARDIO

Makes 12 cups

Prep time: 5 mins
Cook time: 1 min, plus 2 hrs to chill

The ultimate in quick and easy high-fat snacks, these tasty little treats will keep you energized through long cardio workouts. They're so easy to make I encourage all my clients to have a batch on hand in the freezer for quick fuel or for when a sweet craving hits. I use refined coconut oil here to keep the flavor neutral, but you can use virgin if you like a more intense coconut flavor.

½ cup refined coconut oil
½ cup unsweetened creamy peanut butter or almond butter

¼ cup sugar-free chocolate chips

2 tablespoons unsweetened cocoa powder
¼ teaspoon kosher salt

1. Line a 12-cup muffin tin with paper liners.
2. In a microwave-safe bowl, combine the oil, peanut butter, and chocolate chips. (I like to use a glass measuring cup to make pouring into the muffin liners easy.) Microwave on high for 45 to 60 seconds, or until melted. Stir until creamy.
3. Add the cocoa powder and salt. Stir until well combined.
4. Divide the mixture evenly among the prepared muffin cups. Freeze for 2 hours, or until hard and set.

▶ **STORAGE TIP:** Once frozen, these Chocolate–Peanut Butter Cups can be transferred to a zip-top bag and stored in the refrigerator for up to 2 weeks or in the freezer for up to 3 months.

Per Serving (1 peanut butter cup): Calories: 176; Total fat: 16g; Total carbs: 5g; Fiber: 1.5g; Net carbs: 2g; Protein: 3g
Macros: 82% Fat; 7% Protein; 11% Carbs

Lime–Coconut Cream Pops

OVERALL FITNESS

Makes 4 pops

Prep time: 15 mins, plus 6 hrs to freeze

The addition of heavy cream makes these pops super creamy, but you can adapt these to be vegan and dairy-free by substituting an additional ½ cup of coconut milk for the heavy cream. If you don't have ice pop molds, simply pour the mixture into 8-ounce plastic cups and freeze according to the recipe.

---

1 (13½-ounce) can full-fat coconut milk
½ cup heavy cream
¼ cup powdered sugar-free sweetener, such as Swerve
Grated zest of 2 limes
¼ cup finely shredded unsweetened coconut

1. In a large bowl, whisk together the coconut milk, cream, and sweetener for 1 to 2 minutes, or until thick and creamy.
2. Add the lime zest and shredded coconut. Whisk until well combined.
3. Divide the mixture evenly into 4 ice pop molds and insert ice pop sticks. Freeze for 6 hours, or until the ice pops are set.

▸ **STORAGE TIP:** These ice pops will store in the freezer for up to 1 month.

Per Serving (1 pop): Calories: 382; Total fat: 34g; Total carbs: 16g; Fiber: 2.5g; Net carbs: 3g; Protein: 3g
Macros: 80% Fat; 3% Protein; 17% Carbs

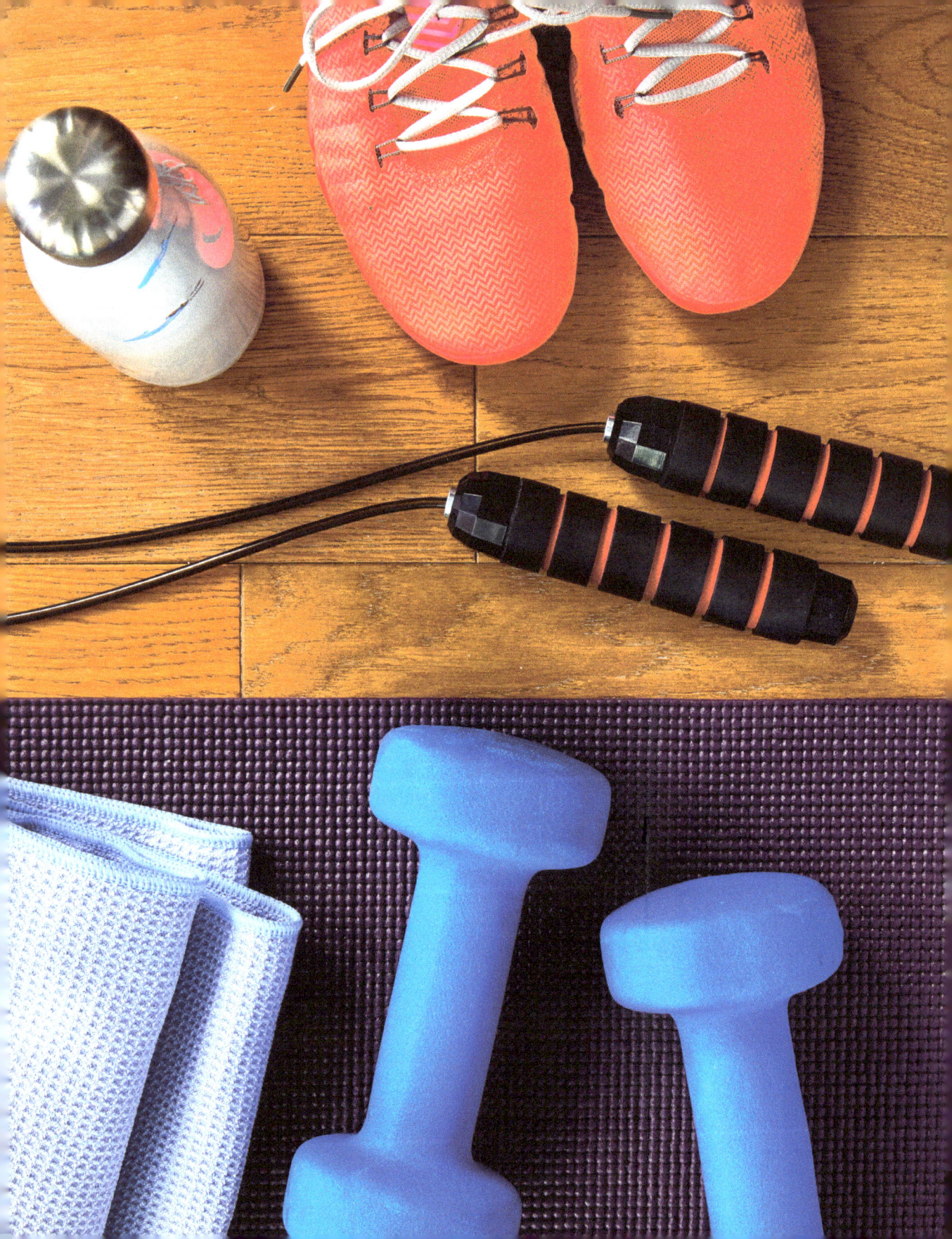

MEASUREMENT CONVERSIONS

VOLUME EQUIVALENTS (DRY)

US STANDARD	METRIC
⅛ teaspoon	0.5 mL
¼ teaspoon	1 mL
½ teaspoon	2 mL
¾ teaspoon	4 mL
1 teaspoon	5 mL
1 tablespoon	15 mL
¼ cup	59 mL
⅓ cup	79 mL
½ cup	118 mL
⅔ cup	156 mL
¾ cup	177 mL
1 cup	235 mL
2 cups or 1 pint	475 mL
3 cups	700 mL
4 cups or 1 quart	1 L

VOLUME EQUIVALENTS (LIQUID)

US STANDARD	US STANDARD (OUNCES)	METRIC (APPROXIMATE)
2 tablespoons	1 fl. oz.	30 mL
¼ cup	2 fl. oz.	60 mL
½ cup	4 fl. oz.	120 mL
1 cup	8 fl. oz.	240 mL
1½ cups	12 fl. oz.	355 mL
2 cups or 1 pint	16 fl. oz.	475 mL
4 cups or 1 quart	32 fl. oz.	1 L
1 gallon	128 fl. oz.	4 L

OVEN TEMPERATURES

FAHRENHEIT (F)	CELSIUS (C) (APPROXIMATE)
250°F	120°C
300°F	150°C
325°F	165°C
350°F	180°C
375°F	190°C
400°F	200°C
425°F	220°C
450°F	230°C

WEIGHT EQUIVALENTS

US STANDARD	METRIC
½ ounce	15 g
1 ounce	30 g
2 ounces	60 g
4 ounces	115 g
8 ounces	225 g
12 ounces	340 g
16 ounces or 1 pound	455 g

REFERENCES

Acheson, K. J., Y. Schutz, T. Bessard, K. Anantharaman, J. P. Flatt, E. Jéquier. "Glycogen Storage Capacity and de Novo Lipogenesis during Massive Carbohydrate Overfeeding in Man." *The American Journal of Clinical Nutrition* 48, no. 2 (August 1988): 240–47. doi.org/10.1093/ajcn/48.2.240.

Campos, H., J. J. Genest, Jr., E. Blijlevens, J. R. McNamara, J. L. Jenner, J. M. Ordovas, P. W. Wilson, and E. J. Schaefer. "Low Density Lipoprotein Particle Size and Coronary Artery Disease." *Arteriosclerosis and Thrombosis: A Journal of Vascular Biology* 12 (1992): 187–95. doi.org/10.1161/01.ATV.12.2.187.

D'Abbondanza, Marco, Stefano Ministrini, Giacomo Pucci, Elisa Nulli Migliola, Eva-Edvige Martorelli, Vito Gandolfo, Donatella Siepi, Graziana Lupattelli, and Gaetano Vaudo. "Very Low-Carbohydrate Ketogenic Diet for the Treatment of Severe Obesity and Associated Non-Alcoholic Fatty Liver Disease: The Role of Sex Differences." *Nutrients* 12, no. 9 (2020): 2748. doi.org/10.3390/nu12092748.

Fontana, Luigi, Samuel Klein, John O. Holloszy, and Bhartur N. Premachandra. "Effect of Long-Term Calorie Restriction with Adequate Protein and Micronutrients on Thyroid Hormones." *The Journal of Clinical Endocrinology and Metabolism* 91, no. 8 (August 2006): 3232–35. doi.org/10.1210/jc.2006-0328.

Gasior, Macieg, Michael A. Rogawski, and Adam L. Hartman. "Neuroprotective and Disease-Modifying Effects of the Ketogenic Diet." *Behavioural Pharmacology* 17, no. 5–6 (September 2006): 431–39. doi.org/10.1097/00008877-200609000-00009.

Gropper, Sareen S., Jack L. Smith, and James L. Groff. *Advanced Nutrition and Human Metabolism*. 5th ed. Belmont, California: Wadsworth, 2008.

Jacob, Aglaee. "Does Eating a Low-Carb Diet Affect Bowel Movements?" *Livestrong.com*. Accessed May 18, 2021. Livestrong.com/article/509998-do-low-carbs-affect-bowel-movements.

Kerksick, Chad M., Shawn Arent, Brad J. Schoenfeld, Jeffrey R. Stout, Bill Campbell, Colin D. Wilborn, Lem Taylor, et. al. "International Society of Sports Nutrition Position Stand: Nutrient Timing." *Journal of the International Society of Sports Nutrition* 14 (2017): 33. doi.org/10.1186/s12970-017-0189-4.

Kosinski, Christophe, and François R. Jornayvaz. "Effects of Ketogenic Diets on Cardiovascular Risk Factors: Evidence from Animal and Human Studies." *Nutrients* 9, no. 5 (2017): 517. doi.org/10.3390/nu9050517.

Mavropoulos, John C., William S. Yancy, Juanita Hepburn, and Eric C. Westman. "The Effects of a Low-Carbohydrate, Ketogenic Diet on the Polycystic Ovary Syndrome: A Pilot Study." *Nutrition & Metabolism* 2 (2005): 35. doi.org/10.1186/1743-7075-2-35.

Mobbs, Charles V., Jason Mastaitis, Fumiko Isoda, and Michal Poplawski. "Treatment of Diabetes and Diabetic Complications with a Ketogenic Diet." *Journal of Child Neurology* 28, no. 8 (2013): 1009–14. doi.org/10.1177/0883073813487596.

Sisson, Mark, and Brad Kearns. *Primal Endurance*. Oxnard, California: Primal Blueprint Publishing, 2016.

Vidali Silvia, Sepideh Aminzadeh, Bridget Lambert, Tricia Rutherford, Wolfgang Sperl, Barbara Kofler, and René G. Feichtinger. "Mitochondria: The Ketogenic Diet—A Metabolism-Based Therapy." *The International Journal of Biochemistry & Cell Biology* 63 (June 2015): 55–9. doi.org/10.1016/j.biocel.2015.01.022.

Włodarek, Dariusz. "Role of Ketogenic Diets in Neurodegenerative Diseases (Alzheimer's Disease and Parkinson's Disease)." *Nutrients* 11, no. 1 (2019): 169. doi.org/10.3390/nu11010169.

Wood, Richard J., Jeff S. Volek, Yanzhu Liu, Neil S. Shachter, John H. Contois, and Maria Luz Fernandez. "Carbohydrate Restriction Alters Lipoprotein Metabolism by Modifying VLDL, LDL, and HDL Subfraction Distribution and Size in Overweight Men." *The Journal of Nutrition* 136, no. 2 (February 2006): 384–89. doi.org/10.1093/jn/136.2.384.

INDEX

A
Alcohol, 15
Arugula Salad, Fuel Up, 60
Asparagus Benedict, 62
Avocados
  Creamy Avocado Dressing, 101
  Guacamole Salad, 64
  Nigiri-Inspired Salmon and Avocado, 74

B
Bacon-Egg Salad, Creamy, 53
Bagels, Keto, 100
Beef
  Braised Beef Short Ribs, 93
  Corn Bread Taco Pie, 82
  Eggplant Lasagna, 89–90
  Flank Steak with Easy Chimichurri Sauce, 92
  Pesto Steak and Broccoli Foil Packs, 91
  Shepherd's Pie, 87–88
Breakfasts
  Breakfast Pizza, 56
  Broccoli and Cheddar Mini Quiches, 50
  Creamy Bacon-Egg Salad, 53
  Fully-Fueled Protein Shake, 51
  Nutty Baked Oatmeal, 52
  Overnight Smoothie Bowl, 54
  Spinach Shakshuka, 55
Broccoli
  Broccoli and Cheddar Mini Quiches, 50
  Pesto Steak and Broccoli Foil Packs, 91
Brussels sprouts
  Shaved Brussels Hash, 63
  Spiced Chicken Wings and Brussels, 73

C
Cake, Lemon–Poppy Seed Pound, 110
Carbohydrates, 8, 18–19
Cardiovascular exercise, 10–11
  Asparagus Benedict, 62
  Baked Chicken Alfredo with Spinach, 78
  Braised Beef Short Ribs, 93
  Chocolate–Peanut Butter Cups, 111
  Cookie Dough Fat Bombs, 108
  Creamy Avocado Dressing, 101
  Creamy Bacon-Egg Salad, 53
  Guacamole Salad, 64
  Lemon–Poppy Seed Pound Cake, 110
  Overnight Smoothie Bowl, 54
  Shepherd's Pie, 87–88
  Slow Cooker Chicken Tikka Masala, 75
Cashew Hummus, 103
Cauliflower
  Riced Cauliflower and Herb Salad, 66
  Shrimp and Creamy Cauliflower "Grits," 70
Ceviche Salad, Simple, 77
"Cheat days," 14
Cheddar Mini Quiches, Broccoli and, 50
Cheese
  Broccoli and Cheddar Mini Quiches, 50
  Chorizo and Cheese-Stuffed Poblanos, 83
  Keto Bagels, 100
  Mozzarella-Stuffed Pork Loin, 86
  Parmesan Chicken Meatball Casserole, 72
Cherries
  Cherry, Chocolate, and Chia Pudding, 106
  tart cherry capsules, 22
Chia Pudding, Cherry, Chocolate, and, 106
Chicken
  Baked Chicken Alfredo with Spinach, 78
  Greek Stuffed Chicken Breasts, 79
  Herby Orange Baked Chicken, 71
  Parmesan Chicken Meatball Casserole, 72
  Slow Cooker Chicken Tikka Masala, 75
  Spiced Chicken Wings and Brussels, 73
Chimichurri Sauce, Flank Steak with Easy, 92
Chocolate
  Cherry, Chocolate, and Chia Pudding, 106

Chocolate–Peanut Butter Cups, 111
Cookie Dough Fat Bombs, 108
Dark Chocolate Mousse, 107
Chorizo and Cheese-Stuffed Poblanos, 83
Cinnamon Streusel Cupcakes, 109
Coconut
 Coconut–Nut Butter Power Balls, 98
 Lime–Coconut Cream Pops, 112
Cookie Dough Fat Bombs, 108
Corn Bread Taco Pie, 82
Crave-Worthy Caesar Dressing, 102
Cravings, 14
Cupcakes, Cinnamon Streusel, 109
Curcumin, 21

D

Dairy-free
 Braised Beef Short Ribs, 93
 Cashew Hummus, 103
 Coconut–Nut Butter Power Balls, 98
 Crave-Worthy Caesar Dressing, 102
 Creamy Avocado Dressing, 101
 Creamy Bacon-Egg Salad, 53
 Easy Slow-Cooked Ribs, 84
 Flank Steak with Easy Chimichurri Sauce, 92
 Fully-Fueled Protein Shake, 51
 Guacamole Salad, 64
 Herby Orange Baked Chicken, 71
 Lemon-Tahini Sauce, 96

Molly's Flavor-Filled Mayo, 97
Nigiri-Inspired Salmon and Avocado, 74
90-Second Keto Dinner Roll, 99
Peanut and Lime Zoodles, 67
Pesto Steak and Broccoli Foil Packs, 91
Riced Cauliflower and Herb Salad, 66
Shaved Brussels Hash, 63
Simple Ceviche Salad, 77
Spiced Chicken Wings and Brussels, 73
Thai-Inspired Ground Pork Lettuce Cups, 85
Desserts
 Cherry, Chocolate, and Chia Pudding, 106
 Chocolate–Peanut Butter Cups, 111
 Cinnamon Streusel Cupcakes, 109
 Cookie Dough Fat Bombs, 108
 Dark Chocolate Mousse, 107
 Lemon–Poppy Seed Pound Cake, 110
 Lime–Coconut Cream Pops, 112
Dressings
 Crave-Worthy Caesar Dressing, 102
 Creamy Avocado Dressing, 101

E

Eggplant Lasagna, 89–90
Eggs
 Asparagus Benedict, 62
 Broccoli and Cheddar Mini Quiches, 50

Creamy Bacon-Egg Salad, 53
Spinach Shakshuka, 55
Electrolytes, 22
Equipment, 22–23
Exercise, 9–12

F

Fat Bombs, Cookie Dough, 108
Fats, 7
Fish and seafood
 Fish Tacos in Lettuce Boats, 76
 Nigiri-Inspired Salmon and Avocado, 74
 Shrimp and Creamy Cauliflower "Grits," 70
 Simple Ceviche Salad, 77
Fish oil, 22
Freezer staples, 19–20

G

Gluten-free
 Baked Chicken Alfredo with Spinach, 78
 Braised Beef Short Ribs, 93
 Breakfast Pizza, 56
 Broccoli and Cheddar Mini Quiches, 50
 Cashew Hummus, 103
 Cherry, Chocolate, and Chia Pudding, 106
 Chocolate–Peanut Butter Cups, 111
 Chorizo and Cheese-Stuffed Poblanos, 83
 Cinnamon Streusel Cupcakes, 109
 Coconut–Nut Butter Power Balls, 98
 Cookie Dough Fat Bombs, 108
 Corn Bread Taco Pie, 82

Gluten-free (continued)
  Crave-Worthy Caesar Dressing, 102
  Creamy Avocado Dressing, 101
  Creamy Bacon-Egg Salad, 53
  Dark Chocolate Mousse, 107
  Easy Greek Salad, 65
  Eggplant Lasagna, 89–90
  Fish Tacos in Lettuce Boats, 76
  Flank Steak with Easy Chimichurri Sauce, 92
  Fuel Up Arugula Salad, 60
  Fully-Fueled Protein Shake, 51
  Greek Stuffed Chicken Breasts, 79
  Guacamole Salad, 64
  Herby Orange Baked Chicken, 71
  Keto Bagels, 100
  Lemon–Poppy Seed Pound Cake, 110
  Lemon-Tahini Sauce, 96
  Lime-Coconut Cream Pops, 112
  Molly's Flavor-Filled Mayo, 97
  Mozzarella-Stuffed Pork Loin, 86
  Nigiri-Inspired Salmon and Avocado, 74
  90-Second Keto Dinner Roll, 99
  Overnight Smoothie Bowl, 54
  Parmesan Chicken Meatball Casserole, 72
  Peanut and Lime Zoodles, 67
  Pesto Steak and Broccoli Foil Packs, 91
  Riced Cauliflower and Herb Salad, 66
  Shaved Brussels Hash, 63
  Shepherd's Pie, 87–88
  Shrimp and Creamy Cauliflower "Grits," 70
  Simple Ceviche Salad, 77
  Slow Cooker Chicken Tikka Masala, 75
  Spiced Chicken Wings and Brussels, 73
  Spinach Shakshuka, 55
  Thai-Inspired Ground Pork Lettuce Cups, 85
  Zucchini Tots, 61
Grocery shopping tips, 24
Guacamole Salad, 64

H

Hummus, Cashew, 103
Hydration, 13–14

I

Ingredient staples, 19–21
Intermittent fasting, 13

K

Ketogenic diets. See also Meal prepping and planning
  about, 5–8
  exercise and, 9–12
  fitness goals and, 4–5
  rules, 13–15
Ketosis, 6, 9
Kitchen cleanse, 18–19

L

Lasagna, Eggplant, 89–90
Lemons
  Lemon–Poppy Seed Pound Cake, 110
  Lemon-Tahini Sauce, 96
  Simple Ceviche Salad, 77
Lettuce
  Fish Tacos in Lettuce Boats, 76
  Thai-Inspired Ground Pork Lettuce Cups, 85
Limes
  Lime-Coconut Cream Pops, 112
  Peanut and Lime Zoodles, 67
  Simple Ceviche Salad, 77

M

Macronutrients, 7–8
Mayo, Molly's Flavor-Filled, 97
MCT oil, 22
Meal prepping and planning adjustments, 28
  keto jump start plan, 29–33
  maintenance plan, 41–45
  muscle building plan, 37–41
  tips, 24–25, 29
  weight loss plan, 33–37
Meatball Casserole, Parmesan Chicken, 72
Mozzarella-Stuffed Pork Loin, 86

N

Nigiri-Inspired Salmon and Avocado, 74
Nut Butter Power Balls, Coconut, 98
Nut-free
  Asparagus Benedict, 62
  Baked Chicken Alfredo with Spinach, 78
  Braised Beef Short Ribs, 93
  Breakfast Pizza, 56
  Broccoli and Cheddar Mini Quiches, 50
  Chorizo and Cheese-Stuffed Poblanos, 83

Crave-Worthy Caesar
  Dressing, 102
Creamy Avocado
  Dressing, 101
Creamy Bacon-Egg
  Salad, 53
Dark Chocolate
  Mousse, 107
Easy Greek Salad, 65
Easy Slow-Cooked Ribs, 84
Eggplant Lasagna, 89–90
Flank Steak with Easy
  Chimichurri Sauce, 92
Greek Stuffed Chicken
  Breasts, 79
Guacamole Salad, 64
Herby Orange Baked
  Chicken, 71
Lemon-Tahini Sauce, 96
Molly's Flavor-Filled
  Mayo, 97
Mozzarella-Stuffed
  Pork Loin, 86
Nigiri-Inspired Salmon
  and Avocado, 74
Riced Cauliflower and
  Herb Salad, 66
Shaved Brussels Hash, 63
Shepherd's Pie, 87–88
Shrimp and Creamy
  Cauliflower "Grits," 70
Simple Ceviche Salad, 77
Spiced Chicken Wings
  and Brussels, 73
Spinach Shakshuka, 55
Thai-Inspired Ground Pork
  Lettuce Cups, 85
Nutty Baked Oatmeal, 52

O

Oatmeal, Nutty Baked, 52
Omega-3 fatty acids, 22
Orange Baked Chicken,
  Herby, 71
Overall fitness

Broccoli and Cheddar
  Mini Quiches, 50
Cashew Hummus, 103
Cherry, Chocolate, and
  Chia Pudding, 106
Chorizo and Cheese-
  Stuffed Poblanos, 83
Cinnamon Streusel
  Cupcakes, 109
Crave-Worthy Caesar
  Dressing, 102
Dark Chocolate Mousse, 107
Easy Greek Salad, 65
Easy Slow-Cooked Ribs, 84
Eggplant Lasagna, 89–90
Fish Tacos in Lettuce
  Boats, 76
Flank Steak with Easy
  Chimichurri Sauce, 92
Fuel Up Arugula Salad, 60
Fully-Fueled Protein
  Shake, 51
Keto Bagels, 100
Lemon-Tahini Sauce, 96
Lime-Coconut Cream
  Pops, 112
Molly's Flavor-Filled
  Mayo, 97
Mozzarella-Stuffed
  Pork Loin, 86
Nigiri-Inspired Salmon
  and Avocado, 74
Parmesan Chicken
  Meatball Casserole, 72
Peanut and Lime
  Zoodles, 67
Pesto Steak and Broccoli
  Foil Packs, 91
Riced Cauliflower and
  Herb Salad, 66
Shaved Brussels Hash, 63
Shrimp and Creamy
  Cauliflower "Grits," 70
Spiced Chicken Wings
  and Brussels, 73

Spinach Shakshuka, 55
Thai-Inspired Ground Pork
  Lettuce Cups, 85
Zucchini Tots, 61

P

Pantry staples, 20–21
Parmesan Chicken Meatball
  Casserole, 72
Peanut butter
  Chocolate–Peanut
    Butter Cups, 111
  Peanut and Lime
    Zoodles, 67
Pesto Steak and Broccoli
  Foil Packs, 91
Pizza, Breakfast, 56
Poblanos, Chorizo and
  Cheese-Stuffed, 83
Poppy Seed Pound
  Cake, Lemon–, 110
Pork
  Chorizo and Cheese–
    Stuffed Poblanos, 83
  Easy Slow-Cooked Ribs, 84
  Mozzarella-Stuffed
    Pork Loin, 86
  Thai-Inspired Ground Pork
    Lettuce Cups, 85
Proteins, 7–8

Q

Quiches, Broccoli and
  Cheddar Mini, 50

R

Refrigerator staples, 19–20
Rest, 12, 14
Roll, 90-Second Keto
  Dinner, 99

S

Salads
  Creamy Bacon-Egg
    Salad, 53

Index ◂ 121

Salads (*continued*)
  Easy Greek Salad, 65
  Fuel Up Arugula Salad, 60
  Guacamole Salad, 64
  Riced Cauliflower and Herb Salad, 66
  Simple Ceviche Salad, 77
Salmon and Avocado, Nigiri-Inspired, 74
Shake, Fully-Fueled Protein, 51
Shepherd's Pie, 87–88
Shrimp
  Shrimp and Creamy Cauliflower "Grits," 70
  Simple Ceviche Salad, 77
Smoothie Bowl, Overnight, 54
Snacks, 28
Spinach
  Baked Chicken Alfredo with Spinach, 78
  Spinach Shakshuka, 55
Strength training, 11–12
  Breakfast Pizza, 56
  Coconut–Nut Butter Power Balls, 98
  Corn Bread Taco Pie, 82
  Greek Stuffed Chicken Breasts, 79
  Herby Orange Baked Chicken, 71
  90-Second Keto Dinner Roll, 99
  Nutty Baked Oatmeal, 52
  Overnight Smoothie Bowl, 54
  Simple Ceviche Salad, 77
Stretching, 12
Supplements, 21–22

T

Taco Pie, Corn Bread, 82
Tacos in Lettuce Boats, Fish, 76
Tahini Sauce, Lemon-, 96
Tikka Masala, Slow Cooker Chicken, 75

V

Vegetarian
  Asparagus Benedict, 62
  Cashew Hummus, 103
  Cherry, Chocolate, and Chia Pudding, 106
  Chocolate–Peanut Butter Cups, 111
  Cinnamon Streusel Cupcakes, 109
  Cookie Dough Fat Bombs, 108
  Creamy Avocado Dressing, 101
  Dark Chocolate Mousse, 107
  Easy Greek Salad, 65
  Fuel Up Arugula Salad, 60
  Guacamole Salad, 64
  Keto Bagels, 100
  Lemon–Poppy Seed Pound Cake, 110
  Lemon-Tahini Sauce, 96
  Lime-Coconut Cream Pops, 112
  Molly's Flavor-Filled Mayo, 97
  90-Second Keto Dinner Roll, 99
  Nutty Baked Oatmeal, 52
  Overnight Smoothie Bowl, 54
  Peanut and Lime Zoodles, 67
  Riced Cauliflower and Herb Salad, 66
  Spinach Shakshuka, 55
  Zucchini Tots, 61

Z

Zucchini
  Peanut and Lime Zoodles, 67
  Zucchini Tots, 61

Acknowledgments

A life of loving sport, competition, good food, and optimizing nutrition is the inspiration behind this book. I am grateful for my parents, who helped me develop all of those passions, as well as my family of athletes, colleagues, and clients I have met along the way.

Brent, Harper, Luke, and Evan, thank you for recognizing that I need my "me" time in the pool or on the trails and knowing we are all happier for it!

And a huge thank you to my fantastic editor, Maxine Marshall, and the whole team at Callisto Media, who make the writing process seamless and fun. I am grateful to have had you by my side during this project.

About the Author

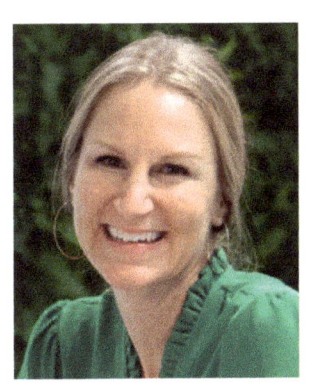

MOLLY DEVINE, RD, is a registered dietitian who specializes in digestive health, healthy weight management, and chronic disease prevention through integrative and functional nutrition. She is an advocate for sustainable lifestyle change through nutrition intervention and founder of MSD Nutrition Consulting, a nutrition counseling and individualized meal-planning service focusing on customized whole foods–based diets for disease prevention and management. She utilizes insurance-based telehealth to work with clients across the country on their health and nutrition goals. Find out more at MSDNutrition.com.

Molly is the author of *Anti-Inflammatory Keto Cookbook*, *Essential Ketogenic Mediterranean Diet Cookbook*, *The Natural Candida Cleanse*, and *30-Minute Vegiterranean Cookbook*. She is also a regular nutrition-focused contributor to online media such as *Shape* magazine, *Insider*, *Greatist*, *HuffPost*, *Brides* magazine, and ABC11 Eyewitness News.

Molly received her bachelor of science in Nutrition Sciences from North Carolina Central University and completed her dietetic internship through Meredith College. She also holds a bachelor of science in Languages and Linguistics from Georgetown University. She lives in Durham, North Carolina, with her family.

CPSIA information can be obtained
at www.ICGtesting.com
Printed in the USA
JSHW031230020921
18359JS00006B/212

9 781648 768941